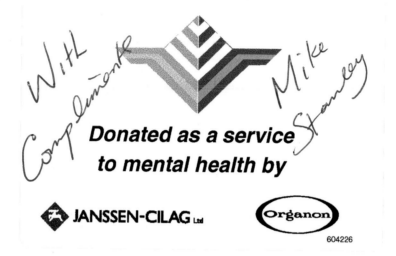

With Compliments

Mike Stanley

Donated as a service
to mental health by

JANSSEN-CILAG Ltd   Organon

604226

ABC OF MENTAL HEALTH

ABC OF MENTAL HEALTH

edited by

TEIFION DAVIES

Senior Lecturer in Community Psychiatry
Division of Psychiatry and Psychology, UMDS Guy's and St Thomas's Hospitals, London
Consultant Psychiatrist
Lambeth Healthcare NHS Trust, London

and

T K J CRAIG

Professor of Community Psychiatry
Division of Psychiatry and Psychology, UMDS Guy's and St Thomas's Hospitals, London

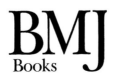

© BMJ Books 1998
BMJ Books is an imprint of the BMJ Publishing Group

First published in 1998
by BMJ Books, BMA House, Tavistock Square, London WC1H 9JR

British Library Cataloguing in Publication Data

A catalogue record for this book is available from the British Library

ISBN 0-7279-1220-8

Typeset by Apek Typesetters, Nailsea, Bristol
Printed and bound by Craft Print Pte Ltd, Singapore

Contents

CONTRIBUTORS

Mark Ashworth
General Practitioner
Honorary Research Fellow, Department of
General Practice, United Medical and Dental
Schools,
St Thomas's Hospital, London

Zerrin Atakan
Consultant Psychiatrist
Lambeth Healthcare NHS Trust
Honorary Senior Lecturer in Psychiatry
United Medical and Dental Schools, St Thomas's
Hospital, London

John Balázs
General Practitioner
Academic Fellow, Department of General Prac-
tice, United Medical and Dental Schools,
St Thomas's Hospital, London

Ann Barker
Consultant Forensic Psychiatrist
Bracton Centre, Oxleas NHS Trust, Bexley
Hospital, Kent

A P Boardman
Senior Lecturer in Social Psychiatry
Keele University, Staffordshire

T K J Craig
Professor of Community Psychiatry
United Medical and Dental Schools, St Thomas's
Hospital, London

Teifion Davies
Senior Lecturer in Community Psychiatry
United Medical and Dental Schools, St Thomas's
Hospital, London
Consultant Psychiatrist
Lambeth Healthcare NHS Trust, London

Simon Dein
Senior Lecturer in Psychiatry
University College and Middlesex Medical
School, London
Honorary Consultant Psychiatrist, Princess
Alexandra Hospital, Harlow, Essex

Claire Gerada
General Practitioner
GP Coordinator, Consultancy Liaison Addiction
Team (Drugs and Alcohol) in
South East London, Hurley Clinic, London

Anthony S Hale
Professor of Psychiatry
University of Sheffield, Sheffield

Ian Hamilton
Care Programme Approach Co-ordinator
Lambeth Healthcare NHS Trust, London

Allan House
Consultant in Liaison Psychiatry
Leeds General Infirmary, Leeds

A J D Macdonald
Professor of Old Age Psychiatry
United Medical and Dental Schools, Guy's
Hospital, London

Martin Marlowe
Consultant Psychiatrist
South Kent Community Healthcare NHS Trust,
Folkestone, Kent

Soumitra R Pathare
Wellcome Research Fellow
United Medical and Dental Schools, St Thomas's
Hospital, London

Carol Paton
Principal Pharmacist
Oxleas NHS Trust, Bexley Hospital, Kent

Amanda Ramiriz
Professor of Liaison Psychiatry
United Medical and Dental Schools, St Thomas's
Hospital, London

Phil Richardson
Head, Co-ordinated Psychological Treatments
Service
Lewisham and Guy's Mental Health NHS Trust,
London
Chair, Psychotherapy Section, Division of
Psychiatry and Psycology, United Medical and
Dental Schools

Howard Roberts
Consultant in Child and Adolescent Psychiatry
Lambeth Healthcare NHS Trust,
London

David Roy
Consultant Psychiatrist and Medical Director
Lambeth Healthcare NHS Trust, London

Philip Sugarman
Consultant Forensic Psychiatrist
Kent Forensic Psychiatry Services, Maidstone Hospital, Kent

Philip Timms
Senior Lecturer in Community Psychiatry
United Medical and Dental Schools, St Thomas's Hospital, London
Honorary Consultant Psychiatrist, Mental Health Team for Single Homeless People (START)
Lewisham and Guys Mental Health NHS Trust, London

Trevor Turner
Consultant Psychiatrist
St Bartholomew's and the Homerton Hospitals, London

J P Watson
Professor of Psychiatry
United Medical and Dental Schools, Guy's Hospital, London

Karen White
Consultant in Community Psychiatry
South Kent Community Healthcare NHS Trust, Folkstone

PREFACE

Mental health problems are among the most common reasons why patients consult doctors. The majority of these consultations take place in primary care, in the accident and emergency department, or in the outpatient clinics and wards of the general hospital. The *ABC of mental health* gives doctors working in these settings guidance on practical management of mental disorders in an easily accessible format. It provides the essential information needed to recognise and manage significant mental disorder safely and successfully, from detecting symptoms, through choice of treatments, to decisions about when and how to seek specialist advice.

The book begins with an introduction to assessment of a patient's mental health problems, and then deals with the disorders most frequently encountered in particular settings, such as primary care and the general hospital. The major categories of mental disorder are covered next in greater detail, followed by chapters on the main mental health needs of vulnerable groups (elderly people, children, ethnic minorities, homeless people). The final chapters cover broader issues of management: guidance on drug and psychological treatments, the law, and risk management.

Managing mental health problems is a multidisciplinary task. We hope that the book will appeal not only to doctors, but to members of all professions involved in mental health: nursing, social work, counselling, and the law (both lawyers and police). We believe its accessibility will encourage debate, the use of a common language between professionals, and, ultimately, better management of mental health problems.

Teifion Davies
T K J Craig

ACKNOWLEDGMENTS

We thank Dr Trish Groves, *ABCs* editor, for her patience and perseverance over many months, and Greg Cotton, Technical editor, for his expertise in the production of the weekly series in the *BMJ*. We are indebted to two anonymous referees—a psychiatrist and a general practitioner—and we are sure they will recognise many of their suggestions and comments in the text of these articles.

1 Mental health assessment

Teifion Davies

Psychiatry in health care

Psychiatry is a branch of medicine: it deals with those disorders in which mental (emotional or cognitive) or behavioural features are most prominent. The cause, presentation, and course of such disorders are influenced by diverse factors; their symptoms can be bewildering to patients and their relatives; and their management may require social and psychological as well as medical interventions. It is not surprising that this complex situation can lead to misunderstandings of the role of psychiatrists (who are neither social workers nor jailers) and myths about the practice of psychiatry.

The bulk of mild mental disorder has always been managed by family doctors. However, patients referred to psychiatrists are increasingly likely to be managed at home by community mental health services or, if admitted to an acute psychiatric ward, to be discharged after a short stay. Many former long stay patients have been discharged to the community with varying degrees of support and supervision. This book will deal with the principles and practice of managing mental health problems.

Psychiatric assessment

There is a myth that psychiatric management cannot proceed without obtaining an extensive history that delves into all aspects of a patient's life. Diagnosis can take only a few minutes, but time must be spent fleshing out the initial impressions, assessing immediate risks, and collecting information about personal and social circumstances that modify symptoms or affect management and long term prognosis.

Accuracy is achieved by close attention to the pattern of evolution of presenting symptoms and examination of a patient's mental state, supplemented by a small number of specific questions. A complete psychiatric assessment requires a detailed personal history, which, if the doctor is not familiar with the patient, may be built up over a series of interviews. The important point is that such detail comes into play only once the basic problem has been clearly ascertained.

Good interview technique
Interview technique is important in all branches of medicine. A good psychiatric interview comprises a series of "nested" processes of gathering information in which gathering of general information is followed by specific questions to clarify ambiguities and confirm or refute initial impressions.

Open questions—The interview begins with open questions concerning the nature of the present problem, followed by more focused questions to clarify chronological sequences and the evolution of key symptoms. Open questions encourage patients to talk and to concentrate on the present situation and help to establish a rapport.

Closed questions—Specific closed questions (equivalent to the systematic inquiry of general medicine) should follow only once a clear outline of the underlying disorder has emerged. These questions form a checklist of symptoms often found in variants of the likely disorder but not mentioned spontaneously by the patient (such as diurnal variation of mood in severe depression).

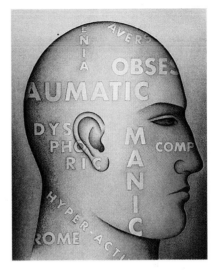

Prevalence of psychiatric morbidity
All mental disorders—>20% of adults at any time suffer mental health problems; 40% of general practice consultations involve mental health problems

Depression (including mixed anxiety and depression)—10% of adults depressed in a week; 55% depressed at some time

Anxiety disorders—3–6% of adults have clinically important symptoms (about 1% each for phobias, obsessive-compulsive disorder, and panic disorder)

Suicide—5000 deaths and more than 100 000 attempts annually; 5% of all years of life lost in people aged under 75 years

Self harm—1 in 600 people harm themselves sufficiently to require hospital admission; 1% of these go on to kill themselves

Schizophrenia (and other functional psychoses)—0.4% of people living at home; 1% lifetime risk; 10 patients on a typical general practice list, but 10 000 not registered with a general practitioner

Bipolar affective disorder—0.5–1% of adults

Personality disorder—5–10% of young adults

Alcohol related disorder—4.7% of adults show alcohol dependence

Drug dependence—2.2% of adults living at home

Anorexia nervosa—1% of adolescent girls

Examples of open and closed questions
Open questions
What are the problems that brought you to see me (to hospital)?
Could you say a little more about them?
And . . .?
Is there anything else you want to mention (worrying you)?
Tell me about your daily routine (your family, your upbringing).
Are there any questions you want to ask me?

Closed questions
When did these problems (thoughts, feelings) begin?
How do they affect you (your life, your family, your job)?
Have you experienced anything like this in the past?
What do you think caused these problems?
What exactly do you mean when you say you feel depressed (paranoid, you can't cope)?
At times like these, do you think of killing yourself?
Do you hear voices (or see images) when nobody seems to be there?

Choice questions
Do you feel like . . ., or like . . ., or like something else?

Choice questions—Sometimes patients are not accustomed to answering open questions. This is often so with adolescents and children, who are more used to being told how they feel by adults. In this case a choice question may be more useful. This suggests a range of possible answers to the patient but always allows for replies outside the suggested range: "Do you feel . . ., or . . ., or something else?"

Initial assessment

The first and most important stage entails getting a clear account of current problems, including social circumstances and an estimate of concurrent physical illness (including substance misuse) that might influence the presentation.

Once the current situation is clear and rapport has been established, closed questions should be used to elicit specific items of history. Topics covered at this stage include patients' prior psychiatric and medical problems (and their treatment), use of alcohol and prescribed and illicit drugs, and level of functioning at home and at work. Initial suspicions of risk to the patient or others should be clarified gently but thoroughly.

> **On each topic the interview should move smoothly from open questions to more closed, focused questions**

Risk assessment—It is a myth that asking about suicidal ideas may lead patients to consider suicide for the first time. Fleeting thoughts of suicide are common in people with mental health problems. Importantly, intensely suicidal thoughts can be frightening, and sufferers are often relieved to find someone to whom they can be revealed. Persecutory beliefs, especially those focusing on specific people, should be elicited clearly since they are associated with dangerousness. Patients who ask for total confidentiality—"Promise you won't tell anyone"—should be reassured sympathetically but firmly that the duty to respect their confidence can be overridden only by the duty to protect their own or others' safety.

Mental state examination

This bears direct analogy with the physical examination and is an attempt to elicit in an objective way the signs of mental disorder. The emphasis is now on the form as well as the content of the responses to well defined questions covering a range of mental phenomena. For example, the form of a patient's thought may be delusional, and the content of the delusions may concern beliefs about family or neighbours.

Physical examination

Relevant physical examination is an important part of the assessment and should follow as soon as is practicable. Usually, this will require only simple cardiovascular (pulse, blood pressure) and neurological (muscle tone and reflexes, cranial nerves) examination. Similarly, laboratory investigations should be performed as indicated, considering a patient's past health and intended treatment. The choice may be influenced by

- Patient's age
- Known or suspected concurrent physical disease
- Alcohol or substance misuse
- Intended drug treatment (especially antidepressants or antipsychotics)
- Concurrent medication (several drugs potentiate the cardiac effects of antidepressants and antipsychotics).

An electrocardiogram is now mandatory before starting certain antipsychotic drugs.

Dos and don'ts in the psychiatric interview

Do

Do let the patient tell his or her story
Do take the patient seriously
Do allow time for emotions to calm
Do inquire about thoughts of suicide or violence
Do offer reassurance where possible
Do start to forge a trusting relationship
Do remember that listening is doing something

Don't

Don't use closed questions too soon
Don't pay more attention to the case notes than to the patient
Don't be too rigid or disorganised: exert flexible control
Don't avoid sensitive topics (such as ideas of harm to self or others) or embarrassing ones (such as sexual history)
Don't take at face value technical words the patient might use (such as depressed, paranoid)

Remember

Put your patient at ease—it is an interview not an interrogation
Be neutral—avoid pressure to "take sides" or to collude with or against the patient

---

Important items of mental state examination

Appearance—Attire, cleanliness; posture and gait
Behaviour—Facial expression; cooperation or aggression; activity, agitation, level of arousal (including physiological signs)
Speech—Form and pattern; volume and rate; is it coherent, logical, and congruent with questioning?
Mood—Apathetic, irritable, labile; optimistic or pessimistic; thoughts of suicide; do reported experience and observable mood agree?
Thought—Particular preoccupations; ideas and beliefs; are they rational, fixed, or delusional? Do they concern the safety of the patient or other people?
Perception—Abnormalities including hallucinations occurring in any modality (auditory, visual, smell, taste, touch)
Intellect—Brief note of cognitive and intellectual function; is the patient orientated in time, place, and person? Is the patient able to function intellectually at level expected from his or her history?
Insight—How does the patient explain or attribute his or her symptoms?

The full mental state examination may be built up over several interviews by elaboration of these topics using increasingly direct, closed questioning.

Tests and investigations

Routine	
Full blood count (including red cell morphology)	These tests should be considered in all patients, but especially in view of:
Electrolytes	Age
Liver function tests	Medical history
Electrocardiogram	Future drug treatment
Urine drug screen	

Supplementary	
Chest x ray	As indicated by presentation or by findings on physical examination.
Skull x ray	
Breath alcohol	They may be needed to confirm or refine the diagnosis, to exclude or define physical comorbidity, to monitor drug treatment
Renal function	
Blood chemistry (eg glucose, thyroid function, drug levels, B_{12}, iron)	
Serology (eg syphilis, hepatitis, HIV infection)	

Special	
Electroencephalogram	These tests should be requested only after seeking specialist advice
Sleep electroencephalogram	
Computed tomography	
Magnetic resonance imaging	
Electromyogram	

Further inquiry

The second broad phase of assessment involves gathering information to place the present complaint in the context of a patient's psychosocial development, premorbid personality, and current circumstances. This phase also follows the scheme of open and then closed questioning, but, because of the breadth of the issues to be covered, it is often the longest component of a psychiatric assessment.

Much of this information may not be available initially, or may take too long to collect in a busy surgery or accident and emergency department. There is no reason to delay urgent management while this information is sought. Similarly, sensitive issues such as a patient's psychosexual history should not be avoided but can be elicited more easily when the patient's trust has been gained.

Making sense of psychiatric symptoms

Although psychiatric symptoms can be clearly bizarre, many are recognisable as part of normal experience. The situation is identical to the assessment of pain: a doctor cannot experience a patient's pain or measure it objectively but is still able to assess its importance. A pattern can be built up by comparing the patient's reported pain—its intensity, quality, and localisation—with observation of the patient's behaviour and any disability associated with it. Similarly, patients' complaints of "feeling depressed" may be linked to specific events in their life, to a pervasive sense of low self esteem, or to somatic features such as disturbed sleep and diurnal variation in mood.

Another myth is that the vagueness of psychiatric features makes diagnosis impossible. In fact, psychiatric diagnoses based on current classification systems are highly reliable. It is true that there are no pathognomonic signs in psychiatry—that is, most psychiatric signs in isolation have low predictive validity, since similar features may occur in several different disorders. It is the pattern of symptoms and signs that is paramount.

In practice, sense may be made of the relation between features and disorders by envisaging a hierarchy in which the organic disorders are at the top, the psychoses and neuroses in the middle, and personality traits at the bottom (Fig. 1.1). A disorder is likely to show the features of any of those below it in the hierarchy at some time during its course but is unlikely to show features of a disorder above it. Thus, a diagnosis of schizophrenia depends on the presence of specific delusions and hallucinations and will often include symptoms of anxiety, depressed mood, or obsessional ideas; it is much less likely if consciousness is impaired (characteristic of delirium, which is higher in the hierarchy). Conversely, personality factors will influence the presentation of all mental (and physical) disorders since they are at the foot of the hierarchy.

Value of the psychiatric interview

The interview is more than an information gathering process: it is the first stage of active management. This may be the first opportunity for a patient to tell his or her full story or to be taken seriously, and the experience should be beneficial in itself. The length of the interview should allow time for intense emotions to calm and for the first steps to be taken towards a trusting therapeutic relationship. The balance between information gathering and therapeutic aspects of the interview is easily lost if, say, a doctor works relentlessly through a pre-set questionnaire.

Some troublesome terms used in psychiatry

Psychosis is best viewed as a process in which the patient's experience and reasoning do not reflect reality. Psychotic symptoms (hallucinations and delusions) may occur transiently in several physical and mental disorders and are not pathognomonic of any disorder. Psychotic disorders are ones that are characterised by psychotic symptoms

Neurosis is a portmanteau term for disorders in which anxiety or emotional symptoms are prominent. It is falling from use since it is difficult to define, has been applied too broadly, and gives no guide to aetiology, intensity, or course

Delusion is a false belief held with absolute conviction and not amenable to argument (incorrigible) or to explanation in terms of the patient's culture. It may be bizarre, but this is not necessarily so

Hallucination is a false perception arising without an external stimulus: it is experienced as real and vivid, and occurring in external space (that is, "outside" the patient's head). In contrast, an illusion is a misinterpretation of a real external stimulus

Confusion is a mild and transient state, in which there is fluctuation in level of consciousness, with impairment of attention and memory

Delirium implies a more severe impairment of consciousness, usually of organic origin, with hallucinations and delusions.

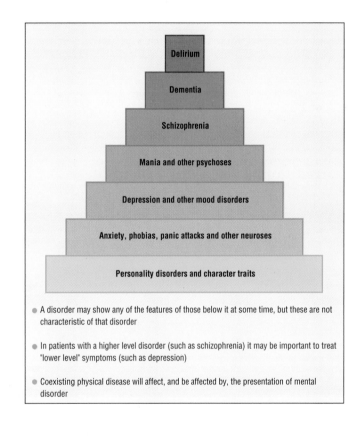

● A disorder may show any of the features of those below it at some time, but these are not characteristic of that disorder

● In patients with a higher level disorder (such as schizophrenia) it may be important to treat "lower level" symptoms (such as depression)

● Coexisting physical disease will affect, and be affected by, the presentation of mental disorder

Figure 1.1   Hierarchy of symptomatology of mental disorders

> For a disturbed patient who is bewildered by his or her bizarre experiences, the interview may be a critical period and the doctor should not waste it

Summarising the findings

A bare diagnosis rarely does justice to the complexity of a presentation, nor does it provide an adequate guide to management. The formulation is a succinct summary of a patient's history, current circumstances, and main problems: it aims to set the diagnosis in context. It is particularly useful in conveying essential information, as when making a referral to specialist psychiatric services. An adequate referral to such services should include

- Description of the presenting complaint, its intensity and duration
- Relevant current and past medical history and medication
- Note of mental state examination
- Estimate of degree of urgency in terms of risk to the patient and others
- Indication of referer's expectations (assessment, advice, admission)
- The most urgent requests should be reinforced by telephone.

Example of referral letter to specialist psychiatric services

Mr A is a 35 year old married man with a three year history of severe depression controlled by antidepressant drugs. He was brought to my surgery by his brother, having tried to break into a church in response to grandiose religious delusions. He also showed irritable mood and pressure of speech suggesting a manic episode. He agrees to attend hospital today. Please assess urgently in view of the risk to himself and others.

Consequences of mental disorder

Patients with mental disorders often suffer *stigma*—the experience of being discriminated against and rejected by others, and a consequent feeling of shame and disgrace. There may also be other serious consequences.

Mortality rates—Psychiatric disorders are associated with increased risk of death from all causes, and the all cause standardised mortality ratio (SMR) among community psychiatric patients is about 1.6 (that is, about 1.6 times the rate in the general population). Mortality rates are highest among schizophrenics (SMR 1.76), men (SMR 2.24), and younger patients (SMR 8.82 for ages 14 to 24 years). Some of this excess is due to suicide and violence, and some to higher rates of respiratory, cardiac, and other diseases. In some surveys, over 50% of patients smoked more than 15 cigarettes per day.

Fitness to drive—A driver with mental disorder has a slightly increased risk of being involved in a road traffic accident, with personality disorders, alcohol intoxication, and side effects of drug treatment accounting for most of the increase. Some disorders (such as schizophrenia, bipolar affective disorder) affect a driver's entitlement to hold a driving licence, at least during the acute illness and for 6 to 12 months afterwards. For other disorders, the period of withdrawal of the licence will depend on the severity of the condition, and may be permanent in some cases (such as severe dementia). Patients have a duty to inform the licensing authority of any such disorder, and the doctor should do this where a patient is unable or unwilling to do so. Care should be taken to warn patients of potential side effects of drug treatment that might affect their driving.

Other aspects—Suffering from mental disorder might affect life insurance premiums, while being detained under the Mental Health Act may restrict a patient's voting rights. Local guidance should be sought in cases of doubt.

Role of voluntary organisations

Several local and national voluntary organisations are concerned with mental health. They may provide telephone advice or support, counselling, day centres, and volunteers or befriending services. Many patients benefit from the counselling or mutual support offered by such organisations, self help groups, and charities. These include patients with severe or protracted mental disorders and their carers, and many others who are distressed by unpleasant circumstances but are not suffering from a mental disorder and so do not require a referral to specialist mental health services.

The artwork is by Sandra Dionisi and reproduced with permission of the Stock Illustration Source. Data on the prevalence of psychiatric morbidity come from government departments, Mental Health Foundation, MIND, MORI, and SANE.

Voluntary organisations offering general help for people with mental health problems

	Telephone No
Carers National Association	0171 490 8898
CarersLine	0345 573 369
Compassionate Friends (bereaved parents)	0117 953 9639
Cruse Bereavement line	0181 332 7227
MIND—National Association for Mental Health	0181 519 2122
National Association of Bereavement Services	0171 247 1080
National Schizophrenia Fellowship advice line	0181 974 6814
Relate National Office (marriage guidance)	0178 857 3241
SANE	0171 724 8000
Samaritans (24 hour emergency line)	0170 875 1111
	0170 874 0000
Victim Support National Office	0171 735 9166
Women's Aid national helpline (domestic violence)	0117 963 3542

Further reading

Department of Health. *The health of the nation key area handbook: mental illness.* London: HMSO, 1994

Kendrick T, Tylee A, Freeling P. *The prevention of mental illness in primary care.* Cambridge: Cambridge University Press, 1996

Kopelman MD. Structured psychiatric interview: psychiatric history and assessment of the mental state. *Br J Hosp Med* 1994;52:93–8

Meltzer H, Gill B, Pettigrew M, Hinds K. *The prevalence of psychiatric morbidity among adults living in private households.* London: HMSO, 1995 (OPCS Surveys of Psychiatric Morbidity in Great Britain, Report 1)

Leaflets

From NHS Executive, Mental Illness, PO Box 643, Bristol BS99 1UU
Mental health: towards a better understanding
Mental health and older people
Can children and young people have mental health problems?
From Royal College of Psychiatrists, 17 Belgrave Square, London SW1X 8PG on various mental health topics
From Department of Health, PO Box 410, Wetherby, LS23 7LN
Contact. A directory for mental health
Contact Update
The Mental Health Foundation, MIND, and the National Schizophrenia Fellowship all produce useful leaflets on various aspects of mental health

2 Common mental health problems in primary care

T K J Craig, A P Boardman

The size of the problem

Psychiatric symptoms are common in the general population: worry, tiredness, and sleepless nights affect more than half of adults at some time, while as many as one person in seven experiences some form of diagnosable neurotic disorder.

These problems are not confined to Western countries. The World Health Organization's study of mental disorder in general health care screened over 25 000 people in 14 countries worldwide and assessed 5500 in detail. A quarter had well defined disorders, and a further 9% had subthreshold conditions. The most common disorders were depression (10%), generalised anxiety disorder (8%), and harmful use of alcohol (3%).

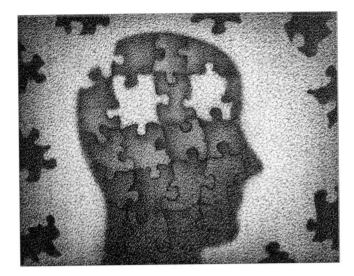

> **Anxiety and depression, often occurring together, are the most prevalent mental disorders in the general population**

The 1993 world development report of the World Bank estimated that mental health problems produce 8% of the global burden of disease, a toll greater than that exacted by tuberculosis, cancer, or heart disease. Much of the burden falls on women and young adults.

Not everyone who experiences symptoms consults a general practitioner, but having a mental disorder doubles the likelihood of consultation. About a quarter of patients with probable mental disorder in the general population will consult in any two week period. People with mental disorders consult more frequently than other patients, and almost a quarter of all consultations are attributable to psychiatric morbidity.

> **Poor outcome is associated with delayed or insufficient initial treatment, more severe illness, older age at onset, comorbid physical illness, and continuing problems with family, marriage, or employment**

Mental disorders in primary care

The World Health Organization's classification of mental disorders for use in primary care pays more attention to the commoner neurotic disorders, while schizophrenia and the other psychoses are classified according to their course.

Mental health problems in primary care
- Emotional symptoms are common but do not necessarily mean that the sufferer has a mental disorder
- Many mood disorders are short lived responses to stresses in people's lives such as bereavement
- About 30% of people with no mental disorder suffer from fatigue, and 12% suffer from depressed mood
- Anxiety and depression often occur together
- Mental disorder comprises about 25% of general practice consultations—In Britain up to 80% of referrals to specialist psychiatric services come from primary care

Bereavement
Death of a loved one is a distressing episode in normal human experience. Expression of distress varies greatly between individual people and cultures, but grieving does not constitute mental disorder. The doctor's most appropriate response is compassion and reassurance rather than drug treatment. Night sedation for a few days may be helpful, but oversedation should be avoided. Antidepressants should be reserved for those patients who develop a depressive episode

---

World Health Organization's classification* of mental disorders in primary health care

Organic disorders	Mood, stress related, and anxiety disorders	Physiological disorders
F00 Dementia	F32 Depression	F50 Eating disorders
F05 Delirium	F40 Phobic disorder	F51 Sleep disorders
	F41.0 Panic disorder	F52 Sexual disorders
Psychoactive substance use	F41.1 Generalised anxiety	
F10 Alcohol use disorder	F41.2 Mixed anxiety and depression	**Development disorders**
F11 Drug use disorder	F43 Adjustment disorder	F70 Mental retardation
F17.1 Tobacco use	F44 Dissociative disorder	
	F45 Unexplained somatic complaints	**Disorders of childhood**
Psychotic disorders	F48 Neurasthenia	F90 Hyperkinetic disorder
F20 Chronic psychotic disorder		F91 Conduct disorder
F23 Acute psychotic disorder		F98 Enuresis
F31 Bipolar disorder		

* ICD–10 (international classification of diseases, 10th edition)

Mood, stress related, and anxiety disorders

Many mood problems are reactions to distressing circumstances (such as bereavement) and resolve spontaneously: patients with such problems benefit from reassurance and time rather than drugs or specialist counselling. About three quarters of patients with new onset neurotic disorders can be expected to recover within a year, but as many as 20% are still symptomatic after three years (Fig 2.1).

A general practitioner with 2000 patients is likely to see one suicide in a four year period. Recent studies indicate that 15-22% of patients who go on to kill themselves will have seen their general practitioner in the week before their death, and 30-40% will have seen their doctor in the previous month. Those people with past contact with psychiatric services are more likely to contact their family doctor in the period leading up to suicide. An opportunity therefore exists for primary care services to help in preventing suicides, and this may be achieved by improved assessment of suicide risk, liaison with mental health services, and more effective treatment of major depression.

Misuse of psychoactive substances

General practitioners can expect to see patients who misuse all types of substances.

Most alcohol related problems in general practice affect moderate users (that is, men who drink 21-50 units a week and women who drink 15-35 units), but a fifth of adults consume harmful amounts of alcohol. However, recent surveys suggest that fewer than a quarter of general practitioners routinely ask patients about their drinking habits. Studies in Britain have shown that 15 minutes of advice from a general practitioner may reduce alcohol consumption by as much as 15% and achieve up to a 20% reduction in the number of patients with drink problem.

About half of general practitioners in Britain report seeing users of illicit drugs, and many practices offer advice on reducing the risk of HIV infection, safe sexual behaviour, and on needle exchange programmes (Fig 2.2).

Benzodiazepine dependence has often been highlighted as a particular problem in general practice. Typically, a general practitioner with 2000 patients will have 60 long term users of benzodiazepines, of whom 45 will be aged over 60. Most will be women who have been taking the drug for more than five years. There has been a steady decline in prescribing benzodiazepines over the past decade, much of this being due to better practices within primary care.

Psychotic disorders

The more severe mental disorders (such as bipolar affective disorder and schizophrenia) are relatively uncommon in general practice. Most of these patients will be in contact with specialist services, although as many as a quarter will eventually be discharged back to the care of their family doctor. General practitioners have a particularly important role in the shared care (with specialist services) of these patients—monitoring physical health, long term medication, and compliance with treatment.

Common presentations

Most patients with mental disorders consult their general practitioner with physical rather than psychological complaints. The complaint may be of "feeling tired all the time," poor sleep, or of not coping with day to day events. Other behaviour at presentation may point indirectly to mental health problems. These presentations may initially mislead an unwary doctor, and the mental disorder may go undetected and untreated for several months.

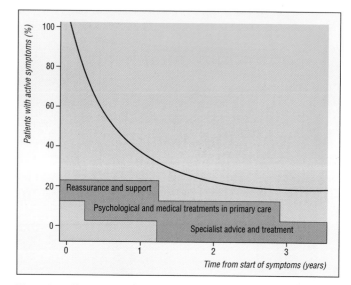

Figure 2.1   Resolution of new onset neurotic disorder and appropriate treatment

Factors that should prompt questions about suicide

Especially if patient is male, single, older, isolated, or shows several factors simultaneously
- Previous suicidal thoughts or behaviour
- Marked depressive symptoms
- Misuse of alcohol or illicit drugs
- Longstanding mental illness (including schizophrenia)
- Painful or disabling physical illness
- Recent psychiatric treatment as inpatient
- Self discharge against medical advice
- Previous impulsive behaviour, including self harm
- Legal or criminal proceedings pending (including divorce)
- Family, personal, or social disruption (such as bereavement, marital breakdown, redundancy, eviction)

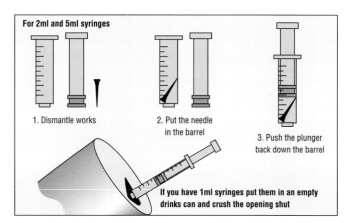

Figure 2.2   Advice to drug addicts on safe disposal of used needles

Mental disorders presenting with physical complaints
- Coexisting physical and mental disorders that are essentially independent of each other (such as heart disease in a patient suffering from depression)
- Distress due to physical illness (such as anxiety or depression related to a life threatening illness)
- Somatic symptoms of a mental disorder (such as palpitations due to anxiety)
- Chronic somatisation disorders in which patients express hypochondriacal convictions that physical disease is present in the absence of any medical evidence for this
- Common physical complaints include
    Tiredness, poor sleep, lack of energy
    Vague aches and pains
    Worry, tension, inability to relax
    Poor memory, "Can't cope"

Detecting mental disorder in primary care

Although the bulk of psychiatric morbidity is seen at the primary care level, only a small proportion of cases is referred on to the psychiatric services (Fig 2.3). In part, this reflects the low rate of detection of mental disorder by general practitioners. Failure to detect mental disorder denies patients potentially effective treatment, and enduring psychological distress has profound effects on patients' capacity to work and enjoy a reasonable quality of life and on their families.

Detection of mental disorder has been shown to reduce the number of subsequent consultations, to shorten the duration of an episode, and to result in far less social impairment in the long term. A doctor's skill in detecting mental disorder has three main components.

Bias towards making psychiatric judgments
Detection of disorder is more likely among doctors who believe that psychological factors play an important role in the aetiology and course of both physical and mental disorder, who express an interest in psychiatric problems, and who believe that mental disorder is an important, legitimate concern of medicine and that mental problems are amenable to treatment.

Vigilance in attending to verbal and non-verbal cues of disorder
Vigilance reflects the extent to which a doctor actively searches for clues about the presence of mental disorder. Many doctors respond with greater vigilance to groups of patients in whom mental disorder is known to be more prevalent (for example, older, female, widowed or separated patients and those who have often attended the doctor's surgery) but miss disorder in patients who do not match the stereotypes.

Quality of interview and diagnostic skills
Neither high bias nor high vigilance necessarily leads to accurate judgments about the presence of mental disorder (doctors with a high bias might overdiagnose disorders). Diagnostic accuracy is not simply related to experience (the number of years in practice) or to the length of time spent with a patient but is rather related to the style and focus of the interview itself.

Doctors with good accuracy ask more open questions, confirm non-verbal cues detected at interview, and inquire about the family and home life of their patients. Patients with emotional disorder, including those who present with somatic rather than psychological complaints, display both a greater number of and more intense verbal and non-verbal cues of mental disorder when interviewed by doctors with good diagnostic skills.

Doctors with low accuracy display interview behaviours that suppress their patients' expression of emotion (closed questioning, narrow focus on symptoms, abrupt manner), which correspondingly lowers the doctors' chances of correctly identifying a mental problem.

Managing mental disorder in primary care

Direct care
Any member of a primary care team may encounter patients with mental health problems and require advice and guidance. A general practitioner's role will include supervising other staff as well as directly managing such patients by means of drugs or psychological treatments.

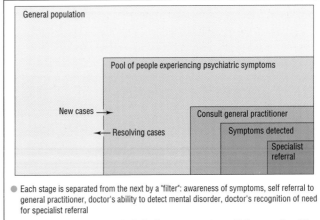

- Each stage is separated from the next by a "filter": awareness of symptoms, self referral to general practitioner, doctor's ability to detect mental disorder, doctor's recognition of need for specialist referral
- The area of each of the rectangles in the diagram represents roughly the proportion of the population affected

Figure 2.3   Stages on the pathway to care

Problems suggesting an underlying mental health problem

Presenting problems
- Seemingly inappropriate requests for urgent attention (appointments, home visits)
- Increased frequency of consultation or requests for tests
- Unexpected or disproportionate outbursts during consultation (tears, anger)
- Excessive anxiety about another family member (child, elderly relative) or presenting a relative as the patient

Recurring problems
- Frequent consultations, "thick notes"
- Unstable relationships or frequent breakdowns in relationships
- Distressing or deteriorating social circumstances (eviction, redundancy, squalor)—Poverty may not cause mental disorder, but it can increase vulnerability and reduce the ability to tolerate symptoms

---

Factors determining the detection of mental disorder

Patient factors
- Nature of presentation (somatic presentation less likely to be detected)
- Severity of disorder (more severe problems more likely to be detected)
- History of psychiatric problems known to general practitioner
- Relatively high frequency of recent consultations

General practitioner factors
- Positive attitude to mental disorder and psychiatric patients
- Interest and knowledge of mental disorder
- "Bias" in assessment
- Interview skills—Doctors who are better at detection
    Make early eye contact
    Clarify presenting complaint
    Avoid "checklist" questioning
    Ask more "open" and clarifying questions
    Spend less time talking and interrupt less
    Seem less rushed
    Show empathy
    Are sensitive to emotional, verbal, and non-verbal cues

In Britain most psychotropic drugs are prescribed by general practitioners, and most moderate anxiety and depressive disorders are entirely and successfully managed in primary care

Although there is insufficient time in the average consultation to undertake formal psychological interventions, many general practitioners who are good at detecting disorder also use psychotherapeutic and counselling techniques to the benefit of patients. Some use double or extended consultations for this purpose. Several studies have found specific interventions by general practitioners to be highly effective.

Other effective interventions include explaining the rationale for treatments, negotiating compliance, checking that advice and treatment are understood, and providing straightforward psychosocial advice on managing distress.

Specialised services in primary care

About a third of general practices in England and Wales have psychological treatment services, most provided by trained counsellors. While there is a wide range of professional backgrounds and therapeutic skills from which to choose, most are based on "non-directive" approaches and psychoanalytical methods. The efficacy of generic counselling (the most common arrangement in primary care) is far from certain as it lacks a strong research base.

We believe that priority should be given to employing staff who can offer treatments of proved efficacy. In primary care cognitive and behavioural therapies are efficient and effective, with proved value in treating depression, generalised anxiety, phobic anxiety (both generalised disorders such as agoraphobia as well as specific fears), obsessive-compulsive disorder, stress related disorder, sexual dysfunction, and the addictive disorders. Nurse behaviour therapists are specifically trained in these techniques but are still relatively few in number. Most clinical psychologists will also be familiar with these interventions.

Patient characteristics influencing general practitioner's decision to refer
- Male sex
- Younger age
- Severe disorder
- Experience of separation in early life
- Associated misuse of alcohol or drugs
- Suicide attempt or suicidal ideation
- Social problems
- Inappropriate responses to medical attention

Effective interventions by general practitioners
- Most moderate anxiety and depressive disorders are managed successfully in primary care
- Brief structured counselling by general practitioner is as effective as anxiolytic drug in generalised anxiety disorder
- No difference in outcome between acute neurotic patients managed by generic community psychiatric nurse or by general practitioner
- Fifteen minutes' advice from general practitioner is effective in aiding reduction of alcohol consumption
- Advice on reducing risk of HIV infection through safe sexual behaviour or needle exchange programmes
- Further examples of general practitioner interventions
  Teaching relaxation techniques
  Supporting use of self help techniques in neurotic disorders
  Supervising withdrawal from alcohol
  Monitoring depot medication
  Operating shared care protocols with local community mental health services

Psychological treatments in primary care settings

Treatment	Practitioner	Programme	Use
Cognitive-behavioural therapy	Nurse therapist or clinical psychologist	6-12 sessions	Effective in depression, generalised and phobic anxiety, obsessive-compulsive disorder, and stress related disorders
Generic counselling using non-directive or psychodynamic methods	Qualified counsellor	Open ended	Used in variety of neurotic disorders Effectiveness not proved
Long term outreach support Case management and other specialist interventions	Community psychiatric nurse	Long term	Effective in patients with severe mental illness Best provided in association with specialist mental health services

Community psychiatric nurses have provided an important link with local specialist mental health services, but their role is controversial. As specialist psychiatric services focus on the needs of patients with severe mental illness, there have been moves to equip community psychiatric nurses with specialised treatment skills for the long term management of this group of patients. These skills include problem orientated case management, family psychoeducation, and psychological interventions aimed at improving compliance (adherence) with medication and coping with persistent psychotic symptoms.

The artwork is by David Ridley and reproduced with permission of the Stock Illustration Source.

Further reading

Desjarlais R, Eisenberg L, Good B, Kleinman A. *World mental health. Problems and priorities in low-income countries.* New York: Oxford University Press, 1995

Goldberg D, Huxley P. *Common mental disorders.* London: Routledge, 1992

Meltzer H, Gill B, Petticrew M, Hinds K. *The prevalence of psychiatric morbidity among adults living in private households. OPCS survey of psychiatric morbidity in Great Britain: report 1.* London: HMSO, 1995

Symposium: prescribing for the psychiatric patient in the non-specialist setting. *Prescribers' Journal* 1996;36:181-228

Pullen I, Wilkinson G, Wright A, Pereira Gray D. *Psychiatry and general practice today.* London: Royal College of Psychiatrists, Royal College of General Practitioners, 1994

Ustun TB, Sartorius N. *Mental illness in general health care. An international study.* Chichester: Wiley, 1995

Leaflets

Bereavement. From: Help the Aged, London EC1R 0BE (telephone 0171 253 0253)

The experience of grief. From: National Association of Bereavement Services, London E1 6DB (telephone 0171 247 1080)

3 Common mental health problems in hospital

Amanda Ramirez, Allan House

The prevalence of mental health problems in patients attending acute general hospitals is high. The three main types of clinical problem are

- Acute primary psychiatric disorder, including deliberate self harm and other psychiatric crises and emergencies
- Psychiatric disorder in patients with physical illness
- Psychologically based physical syndromes (somatisation).

All doctors have a role in addressing the mental health needs of their patients. However, the mental health problems of general hospital patients are closely tied to their physical illness, and specialist units (such as cancer, renal, pain, neurology, or AIDS services) may experience a high level of psychiatric disorder. Patients, and staff, benefit from specific psychiatric liaison support to facilitate integration of their psychological and physical care.

Prevalence of mental health problems in general hospitals

- Hospital attendances for deliberate self harm average 150-200 per 100 000 population. A district general hospital with a population of 250 000 will have about 500 attendees a year. In central London 11% of acute adult medical admissions follow deliberate self harm
- Up to 5% of patients attending accident and emergency departments have only psychiatric symptoms, 20-30% have important psychiatric symptoms coexisting with physical disorder
- Patients with serious physical illness have at least twice the rate of psychiatric disorder found in the general population: 20-40% of all hospital outpatients and inpatients have an important psychiatric disorder
- A quarter of new outpatients to a medical clinic have no important relevant physical disease: 9-12% of referrals of medical outpatients may involve somatisation

---

Key features of a liaison psychiatry service

- Fully integrated multidisciplinary team including liaison psychiatrists, clinical psychologists, psychiatric nurses, and social workers, with special skills in the use of psychological and social interventions
- Based within the general hospital and easily accessible to all departments
- Collaboration with other psychiatric services, social services, and non-statutory services to provide follow up for patients whose continuing needs for care are best met by community services
- Provides a rapid response to immediate problems and emergencies such as deliberate self harm

Features of a service for specialist units

- Initial assessments of patients undertaken jointly by a physician and psychiatrist or clinical psychologist. A model for this approach is the multidisciplinary pain clinic
- Conducts dedicated outpatient clinics alongside the acute specialty clinics
- Provides input to regular psychosocial meetings within specialist units
- Conducts outpatient groups for anxiety and stress management and problems of adjustment to illness

---

Acute primary psychiatric disorder

Deliberate self harm

About 100 000 cases of deliberate self harm present to accident and emergency departments annually in the United Kingdom. Most acts of deliberate self harm involve self poisoning, and nearly half of these involve paracetamol overdose. About 12% of patients injure themselves in other ways, usually by cutting. Alcohol consumption forms a part of about 45% of episodes of deliberate self harm.

Among patients attending hospital with deliberate self harm, the two sexes are currently equally represented and the average age is about 30 years. For most, the act is a response to social and interpersonal problems such as housing or work related problems, unemployment, debt, and conflicts in relationships. Only a minority have severe mental illness.

About 15% of patients attend hospital again within a year of harming themselves and at least 1% commit suicide. In England and Wales about 1000 patients who have deliberately harmed themselves commit suicide each year—almost a quarter of the total annual suicides. The Health of the Nation's target on reducing suicide could be met entirely by halving the suicide rate after hospital attendance for deliberate self harm.

Managing deliberate self harm—Integrated management of such patients is facilitated by overnight admission to an accident and emergency short stay ward, even when this is not medically indicated. This provides the opportunity for adequate psychosocial assessment, including family involvement in the process, and temporary respite from the precipitating crisis. Some patients may, of course, decline admission but should be assessed as fully as possible before they leave hospital.

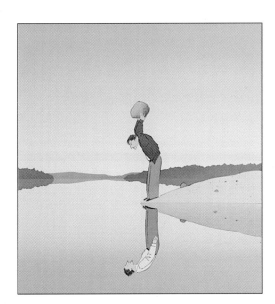

Features of a service to manage deliberate self harm

- Brief admission available to all as an option
- Early psychosocial assessment by specially trained and supervised staff after initial medical management
- Immediate access to psychiatric care where appropriate
- Early follow up by multidisciplinary team, with outreach or domiciliary visits when necessary
- Good communication and liaison with medical and surgical teams, general practitioners, and other agencies

Assessing deliberate self harm—All patients presenting with deliberate self harm benefit from a psychosocial assessment by staff specifically trained for this task. This is in agreement with the Department of Health's recommendations for good practice. The assessment has two functions. Firstly, the sizeable minority of patients who have a psychiatric disorder (usually mood disorder or clinically important substance misuse) can be identified. These patients benefit from standard psychiatric treatment.

Secondly, it provides an opportunity to understand a patient's predicament in a way that integrates symptoms and mental state with information about social and interpersonal difficulties. Full assessment of the context in which an individual episode has occurred improves accurate diagnosis and reduces the pejorative use of diagnostic terms such as "personality disorder."

Intervention after deliberate self harm is intended to improve the social adjustment and personal wellbeing of patients and may reduce the risk of repetition. Brief individual therapy based on a problem solving approach is of most value.

Other psychiatric crises and emergencies

Accident and emergency departments of acute general hospitals are commonly the first port of call for people in crisis. The use of an accident and emergency department by psychiatric patients depends on the organisation of acute general psychiatry services. The proportion of attendees with psychiatric problems is greatly increased if the accident and emergency department is a "place of safety" to which the police may bring a person who seems to be suffering from mental disorder under the Mental Health Act 1983. Many types of acute psychiatric problem may present to an accident and emergency department or occur among inpatients on the wards.

Managing psychiatric crises and emergencies—Assessment of these patients is similar to the approach outlined for patients with deliberate self harm. This can be undertaken effectively by a psychiatric nurse, who coordinates subsequent care with the relevant agencies, including the liaison psychiatrist, general psychiatric services, and social services.

Psychiatric disorder associated with physical illness

Psychiatric disorder may be a consequence of physical illness (such as mood disorder in cancer patients), a cause (such as pancreatitis in patients with alcohol misuse), or a coincidental occurrence. Less than half of the psychiatric disorder in physically ill patients is recognised and treated appropriately.

Mood disorder is mainly anxiety and depression in association with life threatening illness, chronic disability, or hospitalisation. Two thirds of mood disorders tend to resolve as part of the normal process of adjustment to physical illness. A third do not improve unless specifically addressed and so require active treatment.

Alcohol and drug related problems—Alcohol contributes indirectly to many conditions that present to acute general hospitals, particularly gastrointestinal, liver, and neurological disorders. Drug related problems include hepatitis, infective endocarditis, and HIV infection.

Mental disorder may be associated with brain disease (such as stroke, head injury, and epilepsy).

Other psychological problems that may be associated with physical illness include poor compliance with advice or treatment, unexplained handicap, sexual dysfunction, body image disorders, and eating disorders.

Risk groups for deliberate self harm

Patients at high risk
- Those with psychiatric disorder, including
  Major affective disorder
  Substance misuse
  Schizophrenia
- But they constitute only a small proportion of cases

Patients at lower risk
- Those with social and personal problems who are dysfunctional problem solvers due to
  Lack of support
  Previous abuse or neglect
- They constitute a large proportion of cases

Therapy based on problem solving

This includes teaching patients to
- Identify problems and arrange priorities for problem solving
- Generate a wide range of solutions
- Narrow this down to concrete and attainable goals that would represent a personally important improvement
- Work out and implement steps to achieving goals, together with ways of determining and maintaining success

---

Types of acute psychiatric problem that may present in hospitals

- Acute psychiatric disturbance (such as paranoid states, mania, delirium, panic)
- Alcohol and drug misuse, including delirium tremens
- Problems of adjustment to chronic physical illness, especially to repeated hospital admission (such as for asthma or epilepsy)
- Mood disorder (such as anxiety states, depression)
- Personal crises

Identifying psychiatric disorder in physically ill patients

Physical illness with high risk of psychiatric disorder
- Severe, life threatening disease
- Painful, stressful, or disfiguring treatment

Unexplained poor outcome of physical illness
- Poor compliance
- Excessive handicap
- Multiple symptoms or presentations

Patients with high risk of psychiatric disorder
- Previous psychiatric history
- Poor social support

Concurrent psychological symptoms
- Worries
- Anxiety symptoms
- Depressive symptoms

Psychological problems that may be associated with physical illness

- Poor compliance with advice or treatment (such as for diabetes, asthma, sickle cell disease)
- Unexplained handicap, when functional disability after an acute illness is out of proportion to physical impairment
- Sexual dysfunction, which may result from a complex interplay of several factors (emotional impact of the illness, general debility, metabolic and hormonal changes, autonomic and arterial disease, and side effects of prescribed drugs)
- Body image disorders after mutilating surgery (such as colostomy, limb amputation, mastectomy, surgery for head and neck cancer)
- Eating disorders, including anorexia and bulimia nervosa, and obesity (such as in diabetics)

Management strategies for all patients with physical illness

All doctors can act to minimise psychological distress in their patients by

● Identifying worries and concerns (whether accurate or inaccurate)
● Providing factual information and educating patients about their illness and its management
● Encouraging appropriate expression of anxiety and distress
● Reviewing patients to identify any persistent worries and mood symptoms
● Referring patients with persistent psychological difficulties to mental health services.

Treating psychiatric disorder in physically ill patients

The cornerstone of treatment is psychological therapy, either alone or in conjunction with psychotropic drugs. In practice the available treatments are not exclusive and can be modified according to the needs of each patient. For example, in some patients undergoing cognitive-behaviour therapy, an intrusive marital problem may emerge that requires the introduction of marital or family therapy. Psychiatrists must be alert to the development or progression of organic disease and collaborate with the medical team in developing a management strategy.

Psychologically based physical syndromes (somatisation)

Many patients referred to hospital for investigation of physical symptoms do not have an identifiable physical disorder that explains their symptoms. About a quarter of new cases of abdominal pain in gastroenterology clinics and atypical chest pain in cardiology clinics and most general practice referrals to neurology have no relevant physical disease. Many of these patients do not respond to reassurance and, if discharged, are referred to another department or another hospital. Most of these patients have psychological factors underlying their illness.

Somatisation—the presentation of psychosocial distress as physical complaints—has costs to the patients, their relatives, and the health service, particularly in severe and chronic cases. It is associated with a burden of physical and psychosocial disabilities for patients and their relatives. It is costly in terms of unnecessary investigation and treatment, loss of income, iatrogenic problems, and unnecessary welfare benefits.

Psychological treatment of unexplained physical symptoms

There are several psychological approaches to treating unexplained physical symptoms; the better evaluated are based on the principles of cognitive-behaviour therapy.

Clinical characteristics may have a bearing on the particular type of psychological treatment used. For example, markedly abnormal behaviour (such as staying in bed all day) indicates that behavioural treatment might be appropriate (such as graded activity). Cognitive treatment might be better suited to patients with dysfunctional beliefs such as "Investigations should be able to find the cause of my symptoms" or "It is unsafe to do anything on my own."

The artwork is by A Thousand Words and reproduced with permission of the Stock Illustration Source.

Basic psychological skills for all clinicians

All hospital doctors should be able to
● Communicate clearly with patients, discuss concerns, and elicit misapprehensions and correct them
● Break bad news
● Facilitate grieving by patients and their relatives
● Discuss psychological symptoms and distress without embarrassment
● Discuss the need for specialist psychiatric help without seeming dismissive
● Use antidepressants rationally

Treatments for psychiatric disorder in physically ill patients

Brief psychological treatments delivered by trained staff are effective and include grief work, cognitive-behaviour therapy, behaviour therapy, and interpersonal psychotherapy
Non-specific "counselling" and "support" are of limited benefit in managing clinically important psychological problems
Antidepressant drugs are beneficial in patients with conspicuous mood disorder. Tricyclic antidepressants and selective serotonin reuptake inhibitors have similar efficacy but different toxicity profiles. The choice of drug should take account of patients' physical symptoms (for example, tricyclics may benefit those with pain and insomnia but should be avoided in patients with prostatism)

Management strategies for patients with unexplained physical symptoms

It is important that
● Patients' symptoms and their understanding of these symptoms are elicited in full
● Psychosocial cues are identified and explored (such as low mood, distressing events, and personal difficulties)
● Symptoms and investigations are reviewed—Telling patients that "nothing is wrong" is not helpful, but negative findings and their implications should be discussed (for example, "There is no evidence that your symptoms are due to cancer")
● Clinicians then explain to patients that their physical symptoms may have a psychological origin (for example, tension headaches, hyperventilation, and tachycardia may all be manifestations of anxiety). This can be linked to current psychosocial problems that have been elicited
● Management plans can then be reviewed with patients, and limits set on further investigations and drug prescribing
● Revised plans are communicated to the patients' general practitioner to avoid misunderstandings and "doctor shopping"
● Referral to mental health services is considered.

Key references

Managing self-harm: the legal issues. *Drug Ther Bull*, 1997; **35**: 41–3.
Creed F, Mayou R, Hopkins A, eds. *Medical symptoms not explained by organic disease*. London: Royal College of Psychiatrists, Royal College of Physicians of London, 1992
House A, Mayou R, Mallinson C, eds. *Psychiatric aspects of physical disease*. London: Royal College of Psychiatrists, Royal College of General Practitioners, 1995
Royal College of Physicians, Royal College of Psychiatrists. *Psychological care of medical patients: recognition of need and service provision*. London: RCP, RCPsych, 1995
Royal College of Psychiatrists. *The general hospital management of adult deliberate self harm: consensus statement on minimum standards for service provision*. London: RCPsych, 1994

4 Mental health emergencies

Zerrin Atakan, Teifion Davies

An emergency is a situation that requires immediate attention to avert a serious outcome. Mental health emergencies range from situations where a patient is at risk because of intense personal distress, suicidal intentions, or self neglect to those where a patient places others at risk. Some patients may behave in an aggressive manner, make threats, or act violently. Such behaviour may produce physical or psychological injury in other people or damage property.

> In difficult circumstances almost any patient may behave violently and pose a risk to their own safety or that of others

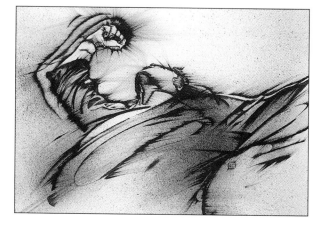

Causes of mental health emergencies

What makes a situation an emergency depends on the individual patient and the circumstances. Surprisingly, patients with mental disorders are more often the victims than the perpetrators of violence. They are often feared by the public, and this may render them vulnerable to assault. A patient's own health is often at risk from his or her behaviour, as in attempted suicide or severe depression. Other people may be more at risk of neglect or accidental involvement than of intentional violence.

Not all emergencies involve psychotic disorders. Neurotic disorders such as acute anxiety or panic disorder can cause chaotic or dangerous behaviour. Misuse of alcohol or illicit drugs may increase a patient's vulnerability, risk taking behaviour, and propensity to violence. The recent increase in suicide rate among young men seems to be due to social and psychological factors rather than recognised mental disorder.

Safety and risk

Preventing violent incidents has two main components—preparation and prediction.

Preparation
This requires constant awareness of potential risks and hazards to personal safety and of the need to maintain a safe environment. The design and layout of the clinic or surgery should be as pleasant and relaxing as possible—patients do react according to their environment. Dead ends, blind spots, and potential weapons should be minimised. All staff should receive regular training in personal safety and emergency procedures.

Dealing with emergencies in the community can be particularly difficult. Just as for medical emergencies, the ability of the lone general practitioner to manage a situation may be limited: the priority is to raise the alarm and obtain assistance without delay.

Prediction
This requires awareness of the risks posed by a specific patient or situation.

Long term prediction—Although its reliability is poor, the best long term predictor of a person's propensity for violence is a history of violent behaviour. Knowledge of a patient's patterns

---

Some mental health emergencies

Immediate risk to a patient's health and wellbeing
- Nihilistic delusions or depressive stupor (stops eating and drinking)
- Manic excitement (stops eating, becomes exhausted and dehydrated)
- Self neglect (depression, dementia)
- Vulnerability to assault or exploitation (substance misuse and many mental disorders)
- Sexual exploitation

Immediate risk to a patient's safety
- Suicidal intentions (plans and preparations, especially if concealed from others)
- Deliberate self harm (as result of personality disorder, delusional beliefs, or poor coping skills)
- Chaotic behaviour (during intense anxiety, panic, psychosis)

Immediate risk to others
- To family (due to depressive or paranoid delusions)
- To children, who may be neglected due to parent's erratic behaviour (in schizophrenia or mania)
- To newborn baby (in postnatal depression or puerperal psychosis)
- To general public (due to paranoid or persecutory delusions or passivity symptoms such as delusions of being controlled by a specific person)

Some important risk factors for violent behaviour
Psychological
- Anxiety or fears for personal safety (attack as means of defence)
- Anger or arguments
- Feelings of being overwhelmed or unable to cope
- Learned behaviour
- History of physical or sexual abuse

Organic
- Intoxication with alcohol or illicit drugs
- Side effects of medication (sedation, disorientation, akathisia, disinhibition)
- Inadequate control of symptoms
- Delirium

Psychotic
- Delusional beliefs of persecution
- "Command" hallucinations to harm others
- Depressive or nihilistic delusions and intense suicidal ideas

Social
- Group pressure
- Social tolerance of violence
- Previous exposure to violence (in home, environment, or media)
The most consistent risk factor is a personal history of violent behaviour

of behaviour, and of what triggers violence, is of greatest importance. This requires careful recording of incidents and clear communication between staff and other agencies.

Short term prediction of violent behaviour depends on recognising the early signs. Threats of violence should always be taken seriously. Worsening of symptoms, especially delusions or hallucinations that focus on a particular person, can be predictive. Other warning signs will vary from patient to patient and may not be reliable. These include changes or extremes of behaviour (shouting or whispering), outward signs of inner tension (clenched fists, pacing, slamming doors), and repetition of previous behaviour patterns associated with violence.

The violent incident

The first consideration in dealing with emergencies, whether violent or not, is the safety of all concerned. Actions taken in good faith to avert imminent disaster are sanctioned by common law and do not require recourse to the Mental Health Act. Formal detention and admission to hospital for continued treatment may be considered later.

Access—Try to obtain unobstructed access to the patient. Clear away movable furniture and potential weapons and ask onlookers to leave quietly.

Time—Do not rush, allow time for the patient to calm down. Most patients can be "talked down" in time. Engaging patients in conversation and allowing them to vent their grievances can be all that is required.

Manner—Talk calmly. Reassure patients that you will help them to control themselves, as aroused patients can be frightened of their own destructive potential. Try to find the cause of the present situation, but avoid heated confrontation. Explain your intentions to the patient and all others present. Be clear, direct, non-threatening, and honest as this will help confused and aroused patients to calm themselves.

Posture—Stand sideways on to the patient: this is less threatening and presents a smaller target. Keep your hands visible so that it is obvious you are not concealing a weapon.

Staff—Trying to cope alone can lead to disaster. Adequate numbers of staff, preferably trained in dealing with such situations, should be available to restrain the patient and contain the incident. In the community, this means summoning help before attempting to deal with a situation. (Fig 4.1)

Medical support—Rapid access to medical services and resuscitation equipment (by ambulance if necessary) should be arranged.

Rapid tranquillisation

Rapid tranquillisation is the short term use of tranquillising drugs to control potentially destructive behaviour. It should be used only under medical supervision and when other, non-pharmacological, methods have failed. In most patients the precipitating symptoms of arousal (tension and anxiety, excitement and hyperactivity) respond to adequate drug treatment in a few hours. (Fig 4.2)

Before administering drugs, ensure that the patient is securely restrained. Injecting a struggling patient risks inadvertent intra-arterial injection (causing necrosis), damage to sciatic nerve (if the buttock is the chosen site), or other injury.

After intramuscular or intravenous administration of drugs, patients should continue to be restrained until they show signs of sedation: further doses might be required. Patients who

---

Emergency admission to hospital

Section 4 of the Mental Health Act in England and Wales
- Permits emergency admission to hospital on the recommendation of one doctor, preferably with previous knowledge of the patient, and a social worker or the nearest relative
- There must be "urgent necessity" (the expected delay if other routes are taken must be stated)

Section 5(2) of the Mental Health Act in England and Wales
- Allows an inpatient to be prevented from leaving hospital on the recommendation of one doctor, provided the patient is under the care of a psychiatrist
- If the doctor in charge of treatment is not a psychiatrist, he or she must act in person (a deputy cannot be appointed) and should obtain a psychiatric opinion as soon as possible

Notes
- It is good practice that these sections be converted to section 2 (which requires the recommendations of two doctors, one of whom must be a psychiatrist)
- If the act is invoked the correct forms must be used and attention paid to detail. It is useful to familiarise yourself with the forms beforehand

---

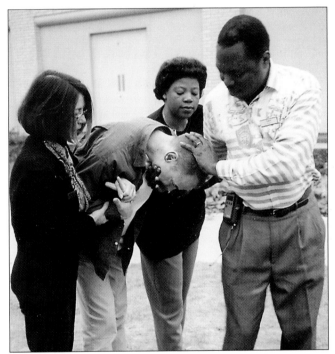

Figure 4.1 Staff practising how to restrain a violent patient without injury

---

Precautions with rapid tranquillisation
- Intravenous administration only under medical supervision: use "butterfly" cannula in large vein
- Administer intravenous drugs slowly
- Ensure resuscitation equipment is available
- If antipsychotic drugs are used, have antimuscarinic drug (such as procyclidine) available in case of acute dystonia
- If benzodiazepines are used, have flumazenil available in case of respiratory depression (give 200 µg intravenously over 15 seconds if respiratory rate falls below 10 breaths/min)
- Use lower dose in
  Older patients
  Patients not previously exposed to drug
  Patients intoxicated with drugs or alcohol
  Patients with organic disorder (delirium)
- Avoid intramuscular chlorpromazine (risk of hypotension and crystallisation in tissues)
- Avoid long acting antipsychotic drugs (including zuclopenthixol acetate) in patients not previously exposed to them
- Avoid antipsychotics in patients with heart disease (use benzodiazepines alone)

accept oral tranquillisation should be allowed to calm down in a quiet room. When sedated, patients should be placed in the recovery position and their heart rate, respiration, and blood pressure should be monitored.

After the incident—aftercare

Everyone involved in a violent or distressing incident, including the patient and any onlookers, may suffer psychological distress. For example, the victim of an assault may go through several phases, being initially numbed or "shocked," later showing anger or emotional distress, and finally succumbing to mental and physical exhaustion. Others may show some of these reactions. Ample time should be allowed for all involved to talk about the incident. Some will be unable to resume work for hours or days. Late sequelae include anticipatory anxiety, flashbacks, and nightmares. Some people may require treatment for depressed mood.

Treating injuries—Any physical injuries sustained during the incident by the patient, staff, or others should be examined and treated.

Recording the incident—The details of the incident should be carefully recorded and reported to the appropriate authority. All services should have specific procedures for this. Staff involved in the incident may require help in recording their involvement.

Involving the police—The police should always be informed if a criminal offence has been committed or weapons have been used. It is usually in the interests of the public and patients to deal with offending behaviour through the courts.

Debriefing—All staff involved should assemble a day or two later to discuss the incident, support each other, and glean any lessons that may be learned.

Suicidal patients

Usually, suicidal patients will talk about their intentions: they should be interviewed sensitively but fully about the frequency and intensity of suicidal ideas and about preparations and immediate plans. Their intentions should be viewed in the context of their current circumstances (precipitating events, losses, social support); history (previous self harm or suicide attempts, known mental or personality disorder); and mental state (depressed, angry, deluded, pessimistic). Those who show clear suicidal intent may need admission to hospital: they should be supervised until their suicidal ideation diminishes in intensity and be given the opportunity to talk of their anguish.

Patients intent on suicide may present a danger to others as well as themselves. They may need to be restrained physically or tranquillised, and all the considerations of safety and follow up mentioned above apply. Profoundly depressed patients, even if showing severe motor and cognitive slowing (retardation), may react with unexpected physical arousal at attempts to intervene.

Major incidents

After a major incident, such as a train crash or a Dunblane-type tragedy, it is now customary to provide counselling for all those involved. This may not be necessary for everyone, but deciding who requires such form of support is difficult in the face of an overwhelming tragedy. Psychological and specialist psychiatric help should be available to those deemed by the emergency services to need it. This will include members of the emergency services themselves. Post-traumatic stress disorder may not be evident for weeks or even months after a serious incident.

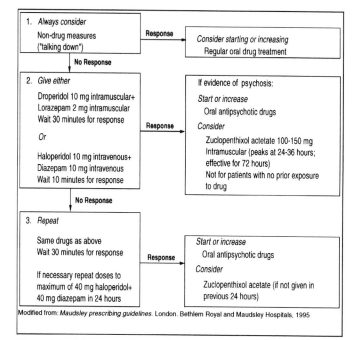

Figure 4.2   Flow chart for rapid tranquillisation of acutely disturbed patient

> Staff may be reluctant to report minor injuries or damage to the police, but their rights to compensation may be compromised if they do not

Further reading

Atakan Z. Violence on psychiatric in-patient units: what can be done? *Psychiatr Bull* 1995;19:593-6.

Cunnane JG. Drug management of disturbed behaviour by psychiatrists. *Psychiatr Bull* 1994;18:138-9.

Pilowsky LS, Ring H, Shine PJ, Battersby M, Lader M. Rapid tranquillisation: a survey of emergency prescribing in a general psychiatric hospital. *Br J Psychiatry* 1992;160:831-5.

Royal College of Psychiatrists. *Assessment and clinical management of risk of harm to other people.* London: RCPsych, 1996. (Council report CR 53.)

Thompson C. Consensus statement. The use of high-dose antipsychotic medication. *Br J Psychiatry* 1994;164:448-58.

Westcott R. Emergencies, crises and violence. In: Pullen I, Wilkinson G, Wright A, Pereira Gray D, eds. *Psychiatry and general practice today.* London: Royal College of Psychiatrists, Royal College of General Practitioners, 1994: 170-9.

The artwork is by Greg Voth and reproduced with permission of the Stock Illustration Source.

5 Community mental health services

Karen White, David Roy, Ian Hamilton

> **Every person with a mental illness shall have the right to live and work, as far as is possible, in the community.**
> **United Nations (1990)**

Community mental health centres should be located in the locality that they serve and provide the base from which multidisciplinary teams deliver the bulk of mental health services for a particular community (Fig 5.1). A multidisciplinary team may include psychiatrists, nurses, occupational therapists, psychologists, social workers, and counsellors supported by an administrative team. The psychiatrist is the bridge between inpatient and community teams and maintains close links with general practitioners, social services, and voluntary organisations.

Who to refer?

When a referral is considered it is important to remember that mental health services are required to focus on the needs of those with serious mental health problems.

Those in distress in the absence of a mental disorder may be helped in one of several other ways: consultation with their general practitioner is all that is necessary for many people with distressing but brief emotional upsets. Assessment and treatment of mild to moderate depressive disorder should also be undertaken by general practitioners. Other patients may be given advice on self help techniques (such as commercially available relaxation tapes) or referred to a counsellor based in the general practice or to a voluntary counselling organisation.

All patients suspected of suffering from a psychotic illness should be referred for assessment. Similarly, anxiety states, severe mood disorders, phobias, and obsessive-compulsive disorders can be disabling and will often require specialist intervention.

Organisation of community mental health services

Assessment and short term treatment

All patients referred to a community mental health team will receive a comprehensive mental health assessment. The initial assessment may be performed by any member of the team, since all should be skilled in history taking and mental state examination. Standardised interviews should be used to ensure that important details (such as physical illness, medication, or alcohol consumption) are not forgotten.

Patients with difficulties not needing specialised mental health services will be directed elsewhere, while others may require further investigation (such as by the psychiatrist, the occupational therapist, or psychologist). Treatments offered may include behaviour therapy, cognitive therapy, medication, time limited counselling, and anxiety management.

Crisis intervention

Many situations in community mental health work require an urgent intervention: from an acute psychotic episode to a suicide attempt after bereavement. Community mental health teams should aim to respond rapidly to anyone believed to be

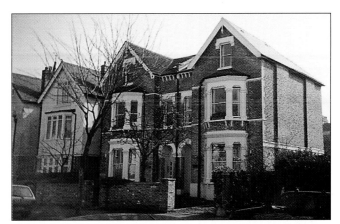

Figure 5.1   Community mental health centre in a suburban street (Lewin Road, Streatham)

Differing characteristics of minor and severe mental disorders

Minor mental health problems
- Brief, time limited, event related
- Sufferers seek help and advice
- May improve with time
- Best dealt with in person's home and family
- Specialist treatment rarely necessary
- Medication usually contraindicated

Severe mental disorders
- Chronic (may be life long) and disabling
- Sufferers often avoid medical contact
- Deteriorate with time if not treated
- Specialist supervision and treatment required
- Medication usually necessary

These represent the extreme poles of a continuum: in the middle are disorders that may be managed by a combination of available resources. When this involves several agencies, the responsibilities of each agency should be drawn up clearly in the care plan.

Advantages of multidisciplinary assessment

- Reduces waiting time for initial assessment
- Ensures attention paid to non-medical aspects of the presenting complaint
  Patients with mental disorders often require psychological or social interventions
  The referring general practitioner will commonly have attended to medical problems or started medication
  Use of standardised assessment interviews by all team members minimises chances of overlooking concurrent physical illness
- Range of treatment options available from early in assessment process
  "One stop" entry to all mental health services
  "Seamless" transfer from one discipline to another

> **The success of community services depends on patients' participation. "Client led" services include patients acting as carers and therapists and being on management committees and appointment panels, and developing advocacy services and employment schemes**

in need of urgent assessment, either at their home or at the mental health centre. For reasons of safety, home assessments of new patients should be performed by two members of the team, and this can prove expensive.

After an assessment of a person's situation and mental state, the team may plan a crisis intervention at the patient's home, admission to hospital (using the Mental Health Act if necessary), or placement in a crisis house if this is available.

At a time of crisis people can be helped to bring about positive changes in their coping strategies—so crisis intervention is appropriate for many psychiatric emergencies. Crisis teams must have immediate support from psychiatrists for prescribing drugs and arranging compulsory admission to hospital.

Other agencies

Successful community mental health care depends on the availability of a wide range of services. Patients need good general medical care and housing appropriate to their level of skill in self care and budgeting.

Social services departments offer advice and social support to those with mental health problems in cooperation with health services. Voluntary agencies may provide day care drop-in centres or counselling and befriending services; others give financial aid or run second hand clothes shops. Self help groups of various kinds provide a remarkable degree of support for many sufferers and their carers. Local liaison and cooperation between all these service providers will make the difference between an ordinary system of care and an excellent one.

Essential elements in a community mental health service

Community mental health centre
- Located in the community to be served
- Easily accessible to patients and their carers
- Services appropriate to needs of local ethnic minority groups
- Multidisciplinary teams which provide
  Crisis intervention
  Non-urgent assessment
  Range of short term treatments
  Long term support of severely mentally ill patients in their own homes
  Long term support of group homes and hostels

Primary care services
- Management of minor mental health problems
- General medical care of those with severe mental illness

User participation
- Patients actively participate in directing development of services

Support from
- Specialist psychiatric (inpatient) service
- Local authority social services
- Local authority housing department
- Voluntary organisations

Cooperation between all agencies facilitated by
- Care programme approach
- Care plans
- Coordination by key worker
- Communication

Key terms in community mental health

Assertive outreach
- Active process in which repeated attempts are made to maintain contact with patients regardless of
  Their location (at home, in a hostel, homeless)
  Their reluctance to receive care
  Their disorganised lifestyle
- Includes actively involving a patient's family and other carers (drop-in centres, day centres)
  To monitor mental state
  To promote compliance with medication
  To improve self care and daily living skills

Key worker
- Mental health worker (such as nurse or social worker)
- First point of contact in a crisis
- Reviews a patient's care plan at regular meetings of patient, carers, and all agencies involved
- Liaises with primary care services, specialist mental health services, and local authority housing and social services

Purchaser
- Usually the local health authority or commissioning agency responsible for implementing public health policy

Provider
- The organisation commissioned by the purchasing authority to provide care to a community (such as an NHS trust)
- The mental health worker who provides care for individual patients

Broker (care manager)
- Health or social services worker who manages a local budget to purchase care for an individual patient
- Under current legislation, such budgets are usually held by local authority social services departments (which then act as care managers)
- Mental health workers may have limited access to these funds, in which case they may act as both broker and provider

---

Severe mental disorder

Services for people with the most severe mental disorders need to be easily accessible to patients and their carers. Traditional care based in large mental hospitals distant from local communities promoted institutionalisation of staff and patients and made no provision for the "assertive outreach" needed to prevent those with the most severe problems from "falling through the net of care."

Closure of many large institutions has significantly reduced the availability of in-patient beds (Fig 5.2), but there is evidence that their former residents have been well served by schemes such as supported housing in the community. However, the needs of large numbers of people with severe mental disorders who have never been mental hospital patients, or those who have lost touch with services, must not be overlooked.

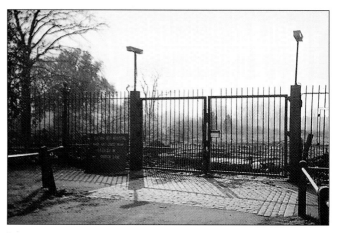

Figure 5.2 Site of the former Tooting Bec mental hospital, South London

Case management

The role of the community psychiatric nurse has become increasingly specialised to meet the needs of severely mentally ill patients. Many are case managers who provide long term intensive follow up to patients with the most severe mental health problems—these are patients who are vulnerable to repeated relapses of psychotic mental illness, have had several admissions to hospital, and often show poor compliance with treatment.

Case managers give practical help with social security benefits, housing, and family support as well as administering drugs and advising on other means of coping with psychotic symptoms. Case management services use an assertive outreach approach to prevent patients from defaulting from contact with services—they may offer extended hours of working, including evenings, weekends, and bank holidays.

Community outreach

Outreach teams offer less intensive follow up to those patients suffering psychotic illness who are more likely to cooperate with follow up and to need less support in dealing with social security benefits and housing issues. Often contact will centre on administration of depot antipsychotic drugs at the patient's home or at a special depot clinic.

Shifting the focus to severe mental disorders

The NHS and Community Care Act 1991 separated the roles of purchasers and providers of health and social care. The responsibility for developing community care plans for people with complex needs rests with the local authority. With mental health, purchasers are required to ensure that providers focus on the needs of those with severe mental health problems, and this is reinforced by implementation of the care programme approach.

This complements and extends the provisions of section 117 of the Mental Health Act 1983, which sets out the responsibilities of health and social services in providing aftercare to patients detained under certain sections of the act. The final tiers of provision are the supervision register and supervised discharge, introduced in 1994 and 1996 respectively, which apply to a relatively small group of severely mentally ill patients who require supervision to ensure that they receive the care they need.

Care programme approach

Everyone accepted by specialist mental health services, including all inpatients, must have a comprehensive assessment of their health and social care needs (Fig 5.3). Then a care plan should be devised and a key worker appointed to arrange its implementation. For most patients, the care plan will be a course of treatment and the key worker will be the person providing it (for example, a psychiatrist, psychologist, nurse therapist, or psychotherapist). The patient will be discharged from secondary care on satisfactory completion of the care plan (or treatment).

Those with more complex needs require a multidisciplinary approach: the key worker should coordinate care and review the care plan regularly with the patient and other members of the multidisciplinary team. This process includes discharge planning for hospital inpatients and involves general practitioners and social workers. Although not mandatory, a case register of those patients with complex needs helps to ensure that they receive regular multidisciplinary reviews.

Changing role of community psychiatric nurses

Case manager
- Intensive, assertive follow up of small number of most severely mentally ill patients living in the community
- Coordinating all aspects of community care (from social security benefits to medication)

Community outreach nurse
- Less intensive follow up of larger number of mentally ill patients
- Regular contacts centred on administering depot medication
- Referring more complex needs to other agencies

Nurse therapist
- Specialised treatments (usually cognitive or behavioural) delivered in defined programme over relatively short time
- May see patients with wide range of mental disorders

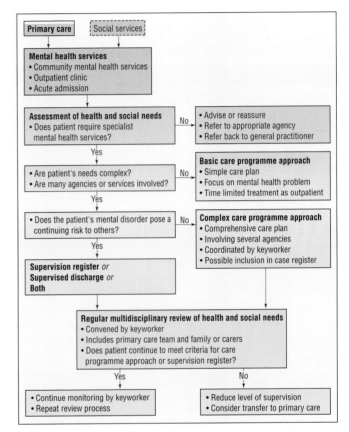

Figure 5.3   Flow chart for developing a community care plan

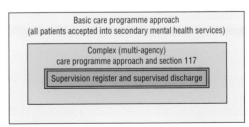

Figure 5.4   Levels of community care planning

Criteria for planning a complex care programme approach

- Patients who, as a consequence of their mental disorder,
    Require involvement and coordination of several agencies
    Have severe social disability or major housing difficulties
- Patients who have suffered repeated relapse of their illness
- Patients who are subject to the aftercare provisions (section 117) of the Mental Health Act
- Patients who are at risk
    Of self harm or suicide
    Of self neglect
- Patients who represent a danger to others

Supervision register and supervised discharge

All health districts are required to maintain a register of patients considered to pose a substantial risk to themselves or others—that is, risk of suicide, severe self neglect, or serious violence to others. The Department of Health estimates that 3000 patients may be included. A care plan should be devised as for the complex (multi-agency) care programme approach, but including a higher level of contact with the key worker and other mental health services (Fig 5.4). In addition to the provisions of the care plan, these patients should have a risk assessment, which may require input from specialist forensic staff. The decision to place a patient on the register rests with the responsible consultant psychiatrist after discussion with the multidisciplinary team.

Supervised discharge is intended for "revolving door" patients—those who may fail to comply with treatment after discharge from hospital and, as a result, pose a serious risk to themselves or others. They will usually be included in the supervision register and receive a similar assessment and services.

Further reading

Department of Health. *Building bridges. A guide to arrangements for inter-agency working for the care and protection of severely mentally ill people.* London: DoH, 1995

Hamilton I, Roy DH. The care programme approach at work in mental health care. *Nurs Times* 1995;91(51):35-7

Kingdon D. Care programme approach. *Psychiatr Bull* 1994;18:68-70

McCarthy A, Roy DH, Holloway NF, Atakan Z, Goss T. Supervision register and the care programme approach: a practical solution. *Psychiatr Bull* 1995;19:195-9

Weller MPI, Muijen M, eds. *Dimensions of community mental health care.* London: Saunders, 1993

Aids to assessing risk

Assessing risk is always a multidisciplinary process. It must take account of

- Patient's history—medical and psychiatric case notes; nursing notes; court reports, witness statements, and other forensic material
- Self reporting by patient at interview
- Examination of patient's mental state and observation of behaviour
- Discrepancies between what is reported and what is observed
- Psychological and, if appropriate, other special investigations

Factors increasing risk of self harm, suicide, or self neglect

Self harm or suicide
- Recent discharge from hospital
- Substance misuse
- Previous self harm or attempted suicide
- Stated intent
- Social isolation
- Recent major life event

Severe self neglect
- Social isolation
- Deterioration after refusing treatment or defaulting from aftercare
- Previous "falling through the net"

Factors increasing the risk to others

Mental state
- Paranoid delusions
- Depressive delusions with ideas of killing others
- Morbid jealousy

Dangerousness
- Threats to repeat violence
- Unwillingness to accept treatment
- Sadistic fantasies

Current episode of violence
- Lack of provocation
- Bizarre violence
- Lack of remorse
- Continuing denial

Circumstances
- Persistence of known provoking events
- Alcohol or drug misuse
- Social difficulties and lack of support

History
- Previous episodes of violence
- Repeated impulsive behaviour
- Inability to cope with stress
- Inability to tolerate frustration
- Diminished self restraint
- Sadistic or paranoid personality traits

6 Anxiety

Anthony S Hale

> **Although there is considerable overlap between the various anxiety disorders, it is important to make a diagnosis as they have different optimal treatments**

Anxiety is an unpleasant emotional state characterised by fearfulness and unwanted and distressing physical symptoms. It is a normal and appropriate response to stress but becomes pathological when it is disproportionate to the severity of the stress, continues after the stressor has gone, or occurs in the absence of any external stressor. Neurotic disorders with anxiety as a prominent symptom are common: a recent British survey found that 16% of the population suffered from some form of pathological anxiety.

Anxiety disorders should be differentiated from stress reactions, in which anxiety may be a prominent feature. These include acute stress reactions—a rapid response (in minutes or hours) to sudden stressful life events, leading to anxiety with autonomic arousal and some disorientation—and adjustment reactions—slower responses to life events (such as loss of job, moving house, or divorce) that occur days or weeks later as symptoms of anxiety, irritability, and depression (without biological symptoms). These are generally self limiting and are helped by reassurance, ventilation, and problem solving. A more profound stress reaction, post-traumatic stress disorder, is described below.

Until recently, the commonest response to a presentation of anxiety has been to prescribe a benzodiazepine. This has been much criticised and alternatives have been evaluated, including almost all the available antidepressants and psychological treatments, especially cognitive behaviour therapy. For most general practitioners, constraints on resources are likely to mean that drugs remain the mainstay of treatment.

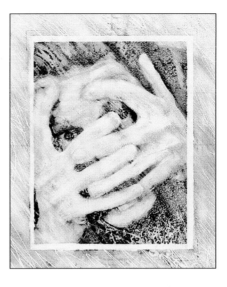

Prevalence of anxiety disorders in adult population*

Disorder	Percentage of population		
	Female	**Male**	**Total**
Generalised anxiety disorder	5	4	5
Phobic disorders	2	1	2
Panic disorder	1	1	1
Obsessive-compulsive disorder	2	1	2
Mixed anxiety and depression	10	5	8

* Data from OPCS 1995 household survey

Classification of anxiety disorders

F40   Phobic anxiety disorder
F40.0   Agoraphobia (with or without panic disorder)
F40.1   Social phobias
F40.2   Specific (isolated) phobias
F41   Other anxiety disorders
F41.0   Panic disorder
F41.1   Generalised anxiety disorder
F41.2   Mixed anxiety and depressive disorder
F42   Obsessive-compulsive disorder

* ICD-10 (international classification of diseases, 10th edition)

F43   Reaction to severe stress and adjustment disorders
F43.0   Acute stress reaction
F43.1   Post-traumatic stress disorder
F43.2   Adjustment reaction
F44   Dissociative (conversion) disorders
F45   Somatoform disorders
F48   Other neurotic disorders
        Includes neurasthenia and depersonalisation or derealisation

Generalised anxiety disorder

This affects 2-5% of the general population, with a slight female preponderance, but accounts for almost 30% of "psychiatric" consultations in general practice. Its onset is usually in early adulthood and its course may be chronic, with a worse prognosis in females. Some genetic predisposition is present, childhood traumas such as separations may confer vulnerability, and it may be triggered and maintained by stressful life events.

This is now regarded as distinct from panic disorder. It is characterised by irrational worries, motor tension, hypervigilance, and somatic symptoms. For most sufferers, it tends to be mild, but in severe cases it may be very disabling.

Diagnosis of generalised anxiety disorder

- Persistent (> 6 months) "free floating" anxiety or apprehension
- Disturbed sleep (early and middle insomnia, not restful)
- Muscle tension, tremor, restlessness
- Autonomic overactivity (sweating, tachycardia, epigastric discomfort)
- May be secondary to other psychiatric disorders such as depression or schizophrenia
- Exclude physical disorders which may mimic anxiety:

Excessive caffeine use	Phaeochromocytoma, carcinoid
Thyrotoxicosis, parathyroid	syndrome
disease	Cardiac dysrhythmias, mitral
Hypoglycaemia	valve disease
Drug or alcohol withdrawal	

Management

Drug treatment

Drugs have been the mainstay of treatment, but the disorder itself is generally chronic, so the potential for tolerance, dependence, and relapse limits the value of anxiolytics to the short term.

Benzodiazepines show a fast onset of action, but tolerance develops with chronic use, leading to increased dose with acute withdrawal reactions on cessation in 30% of cases and chronic reactions in 10%. Side effects include sedation and amnesia and possibly also anxiety and depression: there is substantial potential for misuse and an interaction with alcohol.

Buspirone—Although dependence has not been seen with buspirone, many patients are dubious about its efficacy, perhaps because of its slow onset of action. For chronic anxiety, this is not such a drawback. A trial of up to eight weeks' treatment with at least 30 mg buspirone daily, after gradually increasing the dose for the first two weeks, is often successful.

Antidepressants—Patients who have previously taken benzodiazepines may miss the sedative and acute anxiolytic effects when switched to buspirone, and in such cases a six to eight week trial of antidepressants might be worth while. Antidepressants can produce an initial exacerbation of anxiety, which may be prevented with a benzodiazepine over the first seven to 10 days with little risk of dependence.

The required duration of drug treatments is uncertain, and a common practice is to treat for a similar duration to that offered in depression—six to nine months in the first instance.

Psychological treatments

These are designed to teach skills in managing the cognitive and somatic components of anxiety and are as effective as drugs but with fewer drawbacks. Specialist psychological treatments may be impractical for most patients in primary care, but brief counselling and structured problem solving techniques are effective and may be delivered in general practice. A good outcome after behaviour therapy is predicted by low initial severity of anxiety, while a perception of the outside world as threatening predicts a good response to cognitive-behaviour therapy.

Agoraphobia (with or without panic disorder)

Agoraphobia tends to start between the ages of 15 and 35 and is twice as common in women as in men. Patients suffer acute anxiety attacks when they are in, or anticipate being in, places where escape might be difficult or help might not be available. They have an intense desire to be somewhere else, and their anxiety may be accompanied by the autonomic symptoms of panic disorder. Anxiety inducing situations are avoided, and just thinking about going into such situations may produce anticipatory anxiety.

Management

The efficacy of behavioural techniques such as exposure therapy is well established, and in the long term these may be more effective than benzodiazepines.

Social phobia

Social phobia is a persistent fear of performing in social situations, especially where strangers are present or where the person fears embarrassment. Patients fear that others will think them stupid, weak, or crazy, and exposure to the feared

---

> The efficacy of all treatments for generalised anxiety disorder is best described as modest

---

Management of generalised anxiety disorder

Drug treatment
- Benzodiazepines
  Usually short term use (but watch for tolerance or addiction)
  Long term use in small subgroup of patients (chronic anxiety and long exposure to benzodiazepines)
- Antidepressants
  Tricyclics (not addictive but many side effects)
  Selective serotonin reuptake inhibitors (may exacerbate anxiety initially)
- Buspirone (delayed onset but no dependence)
- β Blockers (block peripheral manifestations of anxiety, especially cardiac)

Psychological treatment
- Reassurance, especially from general practitioner in person
- Counselling and problem solving
- Psychotherapy
  Cognitive-behaviour therapy
  Insight oriented therapy
  Anxiety management (relaxation, breathing exercises, distraction)

> Some patients—especially those with chronic anxiety, a tendency to self treat with alcohol, and a long history of benzodiazepine use—are difficult to manage except with benzodiazepines. When benzodiazepines are used, those with a slower onset of action (not the same as half life), such as oxazepam, may cause less dependence and withdrawal symptoms than diazepam or lorazepam

---

Agoraphobia

Diagnosis
- Anxiety in situations where escape is difficult or help unavailable
- Fear of specific situations, such as
  Alone at home
  Crowds
  Public transport
  Bridges, lifts
- Active avoidance of feared situation, or exposure leads to severe anxiety
- Limitation of functioning (such as shopping, work, social life)

Management
Drug treatment
- Benzodiazepines (short term only)
- Antidepressants (longer term, may exacerbate anxiety initially)
  Tricyclics
  Selective serotonin reuptake inhibitors

Psychological treatment
- Behaviour therapy (especially exposure therapy)
- Group therapy (including self support groups)

situation provokes an immediate anxiety attack. Patients recognise that their fear is excessive, but their anxiety and avoidance behaviour may markedly interfere with their daily routine, work, or social life. Blushing is common, and patients may avoid eating, drinking, or writing in public.

There is some genetic predisposition, onset may follow a particular stressful or embarrassing experience or be insidious, and the disorder usually follows a chronic course. Symptoms often start in adolescence or even childhood and may be associated with poor social or academic performance. The incidence of social phobia is about 2%, but lifetime prevalence ranges from 3% to 13%. In some community studies social phobia is more common in women than men, but the sexes are equally represented in clinical samples.

Management

Only phenelzine and moclobemide have well established efficacy in treating social phobia. Moclobemide is probably the drug of choice, but high doses may be required and treatment should continue for a minimum of three months.

Treatments combining imaginary and actual exposure produce modest gains but seem as effective as more complex regimens. Cognitive-behaviour therapy is promising, either alone or in combination with an antidepressant, but seems most effective in the third of cases with circumscribed social phobias.

Specific (isolated) phobias

This is a circumscribed fear of specific objects or situations. Some community samples have shown an annual prevalence as high as 9% in the general population. Most phobias start in childhood, but situational phobias have a second peak of onset among people in their middle 20s. Particular types of phobias seem to aggregate in families, with some evidence of biological predisposition. Other predisposing factors include traumatic events that affected the patient or were observed in others, and repeated warnings from others about situations. Phobias that persist into adult life usually have a chronic course.

Management

Successful treatment is almost exclusively with behaviour therapy. Drugs are of little use.

Panic disorder

Panic may occur as part of several conditions. However, panic disorder is characterised by unpredictable attacks of severe anxiety with pronounced autonomic symptoms not related to any particular situation. Common features are shortness of breath, fear of dying or of going crazy, and an urgent desire to flee regardless of the consequences.

One year prevalence of panic disorder is 1-2%, with a lifetime prevalence of 1·5-3·5%. Onset is commonest in adolescents or in people in their mid-30s, while onset after 45 is rare. The course of the disorder is variable—sometimes chronic but waxing and waning in severity, or, rarely, it may be episodic. There is evidence of genetic transmission, with first degree relatives of patients at four to seven times greater risk than the general population.

Management
Drug treatment
The choice is between a fast acting benzodiazepine (despite concerns about dependence and withdrawal) and antidepressants, which are well tolerated but have a much slower onset of action. Benzodiazepines are rapidly effective,

---

Social phobias
Diagnosis
- Extreme, persistent fear of social situations
- Fear of humiliation or embarrassment
- Exposure provokes extreme anxiety
- Fear recognised as excessive or unreasonable
- Avoidance of situations
- Anxious anticipation

Management
Drug treatment
- Moclobemide (drug of choice) or phenelzine for at least 12 weeks
- Selective serotonin reuptake inhibitors yet to be proved
- β Blockers used occasionally

Psychological treatment
- Behaviour therapy
    Exposure (in imagination or actual)
    Desensitisation
    Flooding (extreme form of exposure)
    Modelling (therapist demonstrates appropriate behaviour)
- Cognitive-behaviour therapy

Specific (isolated) phobias
Diagnosis
- Extreme, persistent, and unreasonable fear
- Cued by appearance or anticipation of specific object or situation
- Specific objects include
    Animals (spiders, snakes)
    Natural environment (heights, water, storms)
    Blood, injections, injury (may provoke particularly strong vasovagal response with fainting)
- Specific situations—Driving, flying, tunnels, lifts, bridges, enclosed spaces
- Avoidance of situation often with secondary fear of the phobia itself (phobophobia)

Management
- Drug treatment—Minimal response to drug treatment alone
- Psychological treatment
    Behaviour therapy—Exposure, systematic desensitisation, flooding, and modelling (with benzodiazepine treatment if necessary)
    Psychodynamic psychotherapy

Panic attacks

Characterised by acute development of several of the following, reaching peak severity within 10 minutes:
- Escalating subjective tension
- Chest pain or discomfort, palpitations, "pounding heart," tachycardia
- Sweating, chills, or hot flushes
- Tremor or "shakes"
- Feeling of choking, smothering, or shortness of breath
- Nausea, "butterflies," or abdominal distress
- Dizziness, feeling light headed or faint
- Derealisation, depersonalisation
- Paraesthesias
- Fear of dying, loss of control, or "going crazy"

but panic symptoms commonly recur after withdrawal, even with slow tapered discontinuation.

Several older tricyclic antidepressants (such as amitriptyline, clomipramine, and desipramine) and all of the selective serotonin reuptake inhibitors have been found useful in panic disorder at doses similar to those used in depression. Antidepressants often produce an initial increase in anxiety in the first few weeks of treatment before therapeutic benefits appear, leading to poor compliance. This may be overcome by explanation, starting with a low dose with slow increase to therapeutic dose, and coprescription of benzodiazepines for the first one to two weeks.

Monoamine oxidase inhibitors are also effective (for example, phenelzine at doses up to 105 mg/day), and moclobemide may be better tolerated than older drugs. Neither trazodone or buspirone seem to be effective in panic disorder.

Psychological treatment
Cognitive-behaviour therapy and other forms of psychotherapy seem effective against some or all symptoms of panic disorder, with or without exposure treatment. Response to psychotherapy seems to be enhanced by a period of drug treatment to control symptoms. Relaxation therapy also seems to have most benefit when combined with other treatments.

Post-traumatic stress disorder

Anxiety and other symptoms may follow a severe trauma such as an assault or a serious accident. Although formal diagnosis requires an extremely severe stress to occur, similar features are often seen after milder stresses. The relation between the stressor and factors affecting vulnerability, such as personality, is unclear. There is considerable comorbidity with depression and suicide, anxiety states, and other psychosomatic syndromes.

Management

Many treatments have been advocated for post-traumatic stress disorder but with little supporting evidence. Immediate and brief (a few days) treatment with a benzodiazepine may minimise sleep disturbance and mental rehearsal and reduce the chance of chronicity. This should be combined with early debriefing for all concerned. Prolonged symptoms may respond to antidepressants or psychotherapy, or both. One interesting new development for treating flashbacks is eye movement desensitisation and reprocessing (EMDR).

The artwork is by Brad Sherri and reproduced with permission of the Stock Illustration Source.

Panic disorder

Diagnosis
- Recurrent unexpected panic attacks (that is, no specific stimulus)
- Concern about additional attacks (phobophobia)
- Worry about implications of attack (loss of control, "going crazy")
- Change in behaviour related to attacks.

Exclude the following:
- Acute intoxication with or withdrawal from alcohol, caffeine, or illicit drugs (amphetamines, cannabis, cocaine)
- Epilepsy

Management
- Drug treatment
    Fast acting benzodiazepine (alprazolam) in short term
    Tricyclic antidepressants (may exacerbate anxiety initially)
    Selective serotonin reuptake inhibitors (may exacerbate anxiety initially)
- Psychological treatment
    Cognitive-behaviour therapy
    Exposure
    Relaxation is helpful as part of wider treatment plan
- Combination therapy—Ideally, drug treatment should be timed to produce "window" of receptiveness to psychological intervention

---

Post-traumatic stress disorder

Diagnosis
- Exceptional stressor
- Emotional numbness, detachment initially
- Intrusive flashbacks, vivid memories, recurring dreams
- Distress on re-exposure, leading to avoidance of similar circumstances
- Hypervigilance and hyperarousal
- Psychogenic amnesia, insomnia, irritability, poor concentration, distractible, diminished interests, pessimistic mood

Severity affected by
- Premorbid mental or psychological problems
- Repeated similar stress
- Human agency—More severe if stressor caused by another person

Management
Drug treatment
- Benzodiazepines (immediate, short course)
- Antidepressants
- Specialist treatments include
    Carbamazepine
    Clonidine
    Lithium

Psychological treatment
- Debriefing as soon as possible
- Counselling
- Anxiety management (for non-specific symptoms)
- Congitive-behaviour therepy (especially where intrusive imagery and avoidance)
- Stress inoculation
- Assertiveness training
- Group psychodynamic approaches not generally helpful except in cases such as sexual abuse

---

Further reading

Clark DM, Salkovskis PM, Hackman A, Middleton H, Anastasiades P, Gelder M. A comparison of cognitive therapy, applied relaxation and imipramine in the treatment of panic disorder. *Br J Psychiatry* 1994;164:759–69

Hunt C, Singh M. Generalized anxiety disorder. *Int Rev Psychiatry* 1991;3:215–30

Murray M. *Prevention of anxiety and depression in vulnerable groups.* London: Royal College of Psychiatrists, 1995

National Medical Advisory Committee. *The management of anxiety and insomnia.* Edinburgh: HMSO, 1994

Nutt DJ. The pharmacology of anxiety. *Br J Hosp Med* 1996;55:187–91

Shapiro F. Eye movement desensitization: a new treatment for post traumatic stress disorder. *J Behav Ther Exp Psychiatry* 1989;20:211–7

Stopping panic attacks. *Drug Ther. Bull.* 1997; 35:58–62

7   Depression

Anthony S Hale

Depression has a range of meaning—from a description of normal unhappiness, through persistent and pervasive ways of feeling and thinking, to psychosis. Textbook descriptions of depression seen in hospitals are often very different from presentations in primary care.

In recent community surveys, 2% of the population suffered from pure depression (evenly distributed between mild, moderate, and severe), but another 8% suffered from a mixture of anxiety and depression. Even patients with symptoms not severe enough to qualify for a diagnosis of either anxiety or depression alone have impaired working and social lives and many unexplained physical symptoms, leading to greater use of medical services.

Key practical questions relate to treatment. Is any required at all and, if so, what sort and for how long?

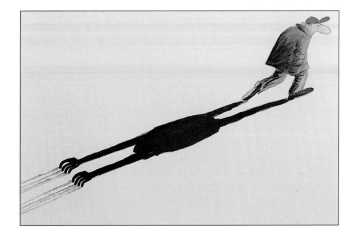

Forms of depression

Most depressions have triggering life events, especially in a first episode. Many patients present initially with physical symptoms (somatisation), and some may show multiple symptoms of depression in the apparent absence of low mood ("masked" depression).

Less severe depression has been awarded many labels, including neurotic depression, minor depression, and reactive depression (not depression as a reaction to circumstances but when reactivity to events in the surroundings is preserved). It is now termed dysthymia, a persistent low grade condition. This may be complicated by episodes of more severe depression, resulting in "double" depression in which resolution of the more severe syndrome is difficult to judge.

Many patients do not fit neatly into categories of either anxiety or depression, and the concept of mixed anxiety and depression is now recognised. The presence of physical symptoms indicates a somatic syndrome (melancholic or endogenous depression). The value of these features in predicting response to treatment is not clear. The presence of psychotic features has major implications for treatment. Brief episodes of more severe depression are also recognised (brief recurrent depression). More prolonged recurrence is now termed recurrent depressive disorder (formerly depressive illness).

Features of depression

Core features
- Pervasive low mood
- Loss of interest and enjoyment (anhedonia)
- Reduced energy, diminished activity

Other features
- Poor concentration and attention
- Poor self esteem and self confidence
- Ideas of guilt and unworthiness
- Bleak, pessimistic views of the future
- Ideas or acts of self harm or suicide
- Disturbed sleep
- Diminished appetite

Somatic syndrome

Present if more than four of the following features are present
- Anhedonia
- Loss of reactivity (loss of emotional reactivity to normally pleasurable surroundings and events)
- Early waking (>2 hours early)
- Psychomotor retardation or agitation
- Marked loss of appetite
- Weight loss >5% of body mass in one month
- Loss of libido

Diagnosis

There are three main distinctions to be made. Is the depression an illness or "normal" unhappiness? If it is an illness, is it a primary psychiatric condition or is it secondary to a physical illness or to alcohol or other drugs? If it is a primary psychiatric illness, is it unipolar or bipolar?

Severity of depression is largely a question of number and intensity of characteristic symptoms. A few mild but persistent symptoms suggests dysthymia. More numerous or more severe symptoms suggest a depressive disorder. Psychotic symptoms (delusions, hallucinations) or depressive stupor are present only in severe depression.

Depression in primary care

- One in 20 visits to doctor due to depression
- >100 depressed patients per doctor's list, but half unrecognised
- 20% develop chronic depression
- Why patients may not mention their depression:

Embarrassed	Avoid annoying doctor
Avoid stigma	Avoid lack of sympathy
Somatisation	

ABC of mental health

Treatment

Much depressive illness of all types is successfully treated in primary care. The main reasons for referring depressed patients to a mental health team are that the condition is severe, failing to respond to treatment, complicated by other factors (such as personality disorder), or presents particular risks. The presence of agitation has been shown to mask psychotic features. Patients with marked psychomotor retardation are also often difficult to treat in primary care.

Medication versus psychotherapy

Basic treatment for mild, moderate, and severe depression and the depressed phase of bipolar illness is generally similar. The principal decision is whether to treat with drugs or a talking therapy. Surveys have shown that most patients in primary care settings would prefer a talking therapy, but evidence of effectiveness is limited to particular forms of psychotherapy.

For mild to moderate depression, cognitive-behaviour therapy and antidepressants are equally effective. For more severe depression, antidepressant drugs are more effective. Cognitive-behaviour therapy is a "brief" focused psychotherapy requiring from six to 20 sessions, and its availability may be limited in some areas. In mild depression patients' response to tricyclic anti-depressants may be no better than to placebo, but this may be related to high levels of non-compliance.

Drug treatment

The use of tricyclic antidepressants at doses well below those that are therapeutically effective (< 125 mg daily imipramine equivalent) has often been reported, especially in primary care. Chopping and changing treatments before giving any one a chance to work (six to eight week trial) is also common.

Effective antidepressant drugs have been available since the 1950s. In the past eight years eight new drugs have been added to those already available—12 tricyclic antidepressants, three monoamine oxidase inhibitors, seven other monotherapy antidepressant compounds, and six fixed combination preparations.

The newer drugs were developed "rationally" to be more selective in their actions than the older antidepressants and hence have far fewer serious side effects than the tricyclics or the monoamine oxidase inhibitors. However, some older drugs—such as desipramine, maprotiline, and nortriptyline—are also selective for noradrenaline reuptake blockade. The differences between drugs lie primarily in their side effects and their potential interactions with other drugs.

Side effects, in particular anticholinergic effects and weight gain, are thought to have a major effect on the frequency with which patients do not take antidepressants as prescribed. Careful clinical studies show large differences between older and newer antidepressants, with much higher non-compliance rates in patients taking the older drugs with more side effects. This merely demonstrates what is clinically obvious—that patients prefer taking drugs with fewer side effects.

Guidelines on the rational prescribing of antidepressants balance their side effect profile, and hence tolerability and compliance, against cost. Economic studies have tended to show little overall difference in costs between drugs, but costs are distributed between many different budgets and it is often difficult for those paying the immediate purchase cost of a drug to take a global view about savings accruing to others' budgets. Clinically, the choice between antidepressants lies in their safety and tolerability to the patient.

Reasons for referral to specialist psychiatric services

- High risk of suicide
- Failure to respond to usual treatment
- Diagnosis is difficult
- Comorbid conditions in which the other illness or its treatment makes treatment of depression problematic (for example, serious physical illness or personality disorder)
- Patients with psychotic depression who may require either combinations of different antidepressants or electroconvulsive therapy
- Patients with bipolar disorder who represent a higher suicide risk during depressed phases and may need careful monitoring of lithium concentrations

> Virtually all available antidepressants are equally effective if given at an adequate dose for a sufficient period

Choice of antidepressant

Tricyclic antidepressants
Available since the 1950s, effective and cheap, but all have dose related anticholinergic side effects that limit compliance. They produce variable degrees of sedation, and postural hypotension may cause falls. Often fatal in overdose. Lofepramine is relatively safe in overdose and almost free of anticholinergic side effects

Selective serotonin reuptake inhibitors
Five now available (fluvoxamine, fluoxetine, paroxetine, sertraline, and citalopram). All lack sedation and are free of anticholinergic effects. This improves compliance but gives less immediate benefit for disturbed sleep (hence, may be combined initially with low doses of sedative antidepressants or hypnotics). All seem safe in overdose. A major benefit with several is that a single or narrow range of doses can be advocated for most patients, usually taken once daily, overcoming the tendency in general practice to prescribe doses of a third to a half of effective therapeutic dose

Monoamine oxidase inhibitors
Rare fatalities from hypertension when taken with foods containing tyramine require a restrictive diet that is unpopular with patients. Traditionally used for "neurotic" or "atypical" depression

Other types
Moclobemide
A reversible selective inhibitor of monoamine oxidase A. Its efficacy is similar to most other antidepressants except, perhaps, in severe depression. An alternative for patients not responding to other agents. Side effect profile is relatively benign, and it is generally not necessary to impose a low tyramine diet. Drug interactions may occur. It seems safe in overdoses of up to 20 g

Nefazodone
A mixed selective serotonin reuptake inhibitor and $5HT_2$ receptor antagonist. Fairly free of gastrointestinal side effects and the sexual dysfunction seen with selective serotonin reuptake inhibitors. More sedative so helps sleep, but some postural hypotension

Venlafaxine
The first mixed serotonin and noradrenaline reuptake inhibitor. It should offer the benefits of tricyclic antidepressants with fewer drawbacks. Side effects are nausea, headache, and sweating. Anticholinergic and cardiovascular adverse events uncommon, and it causes less weight gain than tricyclics. It seems safe in overdoses up to 6·75 g. May cause swings into hypomania in patients with bipolar disorders. Rapid onset of action has been observed

> Non-compliance with antidepressants may reach 50%

Maintenance treatment

Half of all depressed patients only ever have one episode. The risk of a subsequent episode increases with the number already experienced and with increasing age of onset. As risk of recurrence increases, so prophylactic maintenance treatment should be considered, although most patients hate this. There is good evidence of the efficacy of tricyclic antidepressants for up to five years, but few studies of newer drugs extend beyond one to two years. For long term treatment, the burden of side effects with the older drugs is a major consideration in choice of treatment.

Dysthymia

Recently, research has led to a change in the concept of persistent low grade depression from personality disorder to chronic affective disorder.

Past treatment with anxiolytics has now changed to that used in other forms of depression, and there is evidence that most types of antidepressant are effective. However, dysthymic patients may be more sensitive to the side effects of tricyclic antidepressants than those with more severe depression, and hence newer antidepressants may be the treatment of choice. The chronic nature of dysthymia may require long term treatment, particularly when it is associated with episodes of more severe depression (double depression) as recurrence of severe episodes is more likely if the dysthymia is not controlled.

Focused psychotherapies such as cognitive-behaviour therapy and marital and family therapies benefit social functioning but have less effect on symptoms. The marked social and interpersonal debility associated with dysthymia and patients' need to acquire coping skills in managing symptoms and problems suggest that an approach combining antidepressants and focused psychotherapy is most likely to produce lasting benefit.

Psychotic depression

Patients with psychotic depression are the most severely depressed, and they respond poorly to antidepressants alone. Two treatments are effective: combined use of antidepressant and antipsychotic drugs, and electroconvulsive therapy.

Combining some of the newer antidepressants, particularly the selective serotonin reuptake inhibitors, with antipsychotics should be done with caution as inhibition of the liver cytochrome enzymes can raise the plasma concentrations of both drugs, so monitoring may be needed.

Electroconvulsive therapy is an older treatment than antidepressant drugs. It is exclusively a hospital based treatment, and most patients remain as inpatients during the course of treatment. It is effective only for depressed patients who are either deluded or have marked psychomotor retardation. The treatment entails administering an electric charge to the head of a patient under a general anaesthetic in order to produce a generalised fit. From the patients' point of view, they will have a general anaesthetic twice weekly for three to four weeks and experience a mild transient confusional state for an hour or so after each treatment.

Bipolar affective disorder

The clinical features and treatment of the depressive phase of this illness are identical to those of other depressions, but watch for drug induced swings into mania. Effective long term prophylaxis may be achieved with lithium (this requires

Duration of antidepressant treatment for major depression

	Age at first episode (years)		
	< 39	40-49	> 50
First episode	6-9 months	6-9 months	Indefinitely
Second episode	6-9 months	4-5 years	Indefinitely
Second episode with complications	4-5 years	Indefinitely	Indefinitely
Third or subsequent episode	Indefinitely	Indefinitely	Indefinitely

Classification of depression*

Primary
Unipolar
- Mixed anxiety and depressive disorder—With prominent anxiety
- Depressive episode—Single episode
- Recurrent depressive disorder—Recurrent episodes
- Dysthymia—Persistent and mild ("depressive personality")

Bipolar
- Bipolar affective disorder—With manic episodes ("manic depression")
- Cyclothymia—Persistent instability of mood

Other primary
- Seasonal affective disorder
- Brief recurrent depression

Secondary
May be secondary to medical condition or alcohol or other drugs

Depressive episode
Each episode may be
- Moderate or severe
- With or without somatic syndrome
- If severe, with or without psychotic symptoms

* ICD-10 (international classification of diseases, 10th edition)

Electroconvulsive therapy in treating depression*

- The greater the number of typical features of depression, the greater likelihood of a good response to electroconvulsive therapy
- Electroconvulsive therapy is particularly effective in treating depression with psychotic features
- Patients who do not respond to antidepressant drugs may respond to electroconvulsive therapy
- It is essential to continue drug treatment with antidepressants after a successful course of electroconvulsive therapy

Safety of electroconvulsive therapy
- There are no absolute contraindications to its use
- It may be a lifesaving treatment in cases of severe depression
- There is no evidence that it causes brain damage or permanent intellectual impairment
- The risk of death is similar to that of general anaesthesia for minor surgical procedures—about two deaths per 100 000 treatments
- Several drugs, including selective serotonin reuptake inhibitors, may prolong the duration of the induced seizure

* Based on *The ECT handbook*. London: Royal College of Psychiatrists, 1995 (Council report CR39)

pretreatment screening of renal and thyroid function) or carbamazepine; these treatments are usually initiated by psychiatrists.

Suicide and deliberate self harm

There are about 5000 suicides each year in England and Wales, of which 400-500 involve overdoses of antidepressants. Deliberate self harm is 20-30 times commoner. Not all people who commit suicide have psychiatric illness, but, among those who do, depression is the commonest illness and 15% of depressed patients eventually kill themselves.

Assessment of risk is thus important and guides treatment. Many older antidepressants are often fatal in overdose, while the newer effective drugs—such as selective serotonin reuptake inhibitors, lofepramine, and others—are safer and should be used with high risk patients.

The artwork is by Claude-Henri Saunier and reproduced with permission of the Stock Illustration Source.

Suicide or deliberate self harm

Features to be assessed
- Motive
- Circumstances of attempt
- Psychiatric disorder
- Precipitating and maintaining problems
- Coping skills and support
- Risk

High risk indicators for suicide
- Male
- Age >40 years
- Family history of suicide
- Unemployed
- Socially isolated
- Suicide note
- Continued desire to die
- Hopelessness, sees no future
- Misuse of drugs or alcohol
- Psychiatric illness (especially depression, but also schizophrenia, personality disorder)

Information leaflets for patients

Bereavement. From: Help the Aged, St James's Walk, London EC1R 0BE (tel 0171 253 0253)
Depression and your sex life. From: The Depression Alliance, 35 Westminster Bridge Road, London SE1 7JB
Down on the farm? Coping with depression in rural areas; a farmer's guide. Available by calling Health Literature Helpline (0800 555 777)
The experience of grief. From: National Association of Bereavement Services, 20 Norton Folgate, London E1 6DB (tel 0171 247 1080)

Further reading

Bridges PK, Hodgkiss AD, Malizia AL. Practical management of treatment-resistant affective disorders. *Br J Hosp Med* 1995;54:501–6
Clinical Resource and Audit Group. *Depressive illness. A critical review of current practice and the way forward. Consensus statement.* Edinburgh: Scottish Office, 1995
Craig TKJ. Adversity and depression. *Int Rev Psychiatry* 1996;8:341–53
Kendrick T. Prescribing antidepressants in general practice. *BMJ* 1996;313:829–30
Paykel ES, Priest RG. Recognition and management of depression in general practice. Consensus statement. *BMJ* 1992;305: 1198–202
Williams R, Morgan G. *Suicide prevention: the challenge confronted.* London: HMSO, 1994

8 Schizophrenia

Trevor Turner

Schizophrenia is a relatively common form of psychotic disorder (severe mental illness). Its lifetime prevalence is nearly 1%, its annual incidence is about 10-15 per 100 000, and the average general practitioner cares for 10-20 schizophrenic patients depending on the location and social surroundings of the practice. It is a syndrome with various presentations and a variable, often relapsing, long term course.

Although schizophrenia is publicly misconceived as "split personality," the diagnosis has good reliability, even across ages and cultures, though there is no biochemical marker. Onset before the age of 30 is the norm, with men tending to present some four years younger than women. Clues as to aetiology are tantalising, and management remains endearingly clinical.

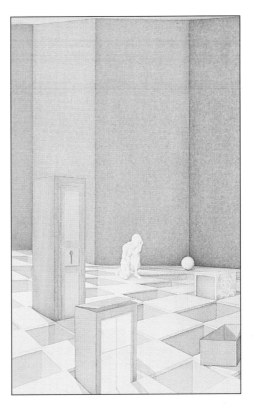

Aetiology

Evidence for a genetic cause grows stronger: up to 50% of identical (monozygotic) twins will share a diagnosis, compared with about 15% of non-identical (dizygotic) twins. The strength of genetic factors varies across families, but some 10% of a patient's first degree relatives (parents, siblings, and children) will also be schizophrenic, as will 50% of the children of two schizophrenic parents.

Premorbid abnormalities of speech and behaviour may be present during childhood. The role of obstetric complications and viral infection in utero remains unproved. Enlarged ventricles and abnormalities of the temporal lobes are not uncommon findings from computed tomography of the brain. Thus, a picture is emerging of a genetic brain disorder, enhanced or brought out by subtle forms of environmental damage.

Clinical features

Positive symptoms and signs

These are essentially disordered versions of the normal brain functions of thinking, perceiving, formation of ideas, and sense of self. Patients with thought disorder may present with complaints of poor concentration or of their mind being blocked or emptied (thought block): a patient stopping in a perplexed fashion while in mid-speech and the interviewer having difficulty in following the speech are typical signs.

Hallucinations—These are false perceptions in any of the senses: a patient experiences a seemingly real voice or smell, for example, although nothing actually occurred. The hallmark of schizophrenia is that patients experience voices talking about them as "he" or "she" (third person auditory hallucinations), but second person "command" voices also occur, as do olfactory, tactile, and visual hallucinations.

Delusions—These are false beliefs held with absolute certainty, dominating the patient's mind, and untenable in terms of the sociocultural background. Delusions often derive from attempts to make sense of other symptoms such as the experience of passivity (sensing that someone or something is controlling your body, emotions, or thoughts). Typical experiences are of thoughts being taken or sucked out of your head (a patient insisted that her mother was "stealing her

---

Symptoms are characterised most usefully as positive or negative, although the traditional diagnostic subcategories (hebephrenic, paranoid, catatonic, and simple) have mixtures of both

---

Clinical features suggesting diagnosis of schizophrenia

- Third person auditory hallucinations
    Running commentary on person's actions
    Two or more voices discussing the person
    Voices speaking the person's thoughts
- Alien thoughts being inserted into or withdrawn from person's mind
- Person's thoughts being broadcast or read by others
- Person's actions being caused and controlled by some outside agency
- Bodily sensations being imposed by some outside agency
- Delusional perception (a delusion arising suddenly and fully formed in the wake of a normal perception)

Note
These features, termed "symptoms of the first rank" by Schneider, suggest a diagnosis of schizophrenia. However, they are not necessary for the diagnosis, and they have neither aetiological nor prognostic importance

---

brain") or inserted into your mind or of your thoughts being known to others (respectively termed thought withdrawal, thought insertion, and thought broadcast). Cult beliefs in telepathy and mind control may relate to partial forms of these experiences.

Negative symptoms

These involve loss of personal abilities such as initiative, interest in others, and the sense of enjoyment (anhedonia). Blunted or fatuous emotions (flat affect), limited speech, and much time spent doing nothing are typical behaviours.

Forms of schizophrenia

Paranoid schizophrenia, the increasingly common form, is dominated by florid, positive symptoms, especially delusions, which may build up into a complex conspiracy theory that seems initially quite credible. The term paranoid has a broader meaning than persecutory, defining a sense of things around you having special, personal significance. Thus, car lights flashing may be evidence that the IRA are following you or proof that a film star is in love with you. The more bizarre the beliefs, the easier the diagnosis.

In contrast, those presenting only with negative symptoms are described as having simple schizophrenia, while hebephrenia is a mix of negative and positive symptoms with insidious onset in adolescence.

The early stages of schizophrenic illnesses can vary considerably. A typical presentation is a family's concerns that a personality has changed or an insistence that a son "must be on drugs." A decline in personal hygiene, loss of jobs and friends for no clear reason, and depressive symptoms mixed with a degree of ill defined perplexity are all common. About one in 10 sufferers commit suicide, usually as younger patients. It is relatively rare for sufferers to assault others.

Classification of the major psychotic disorders*

F20 Schizophrenia

F22 Persistent delusional disorders
Characterised by delusions but without schizophrenia-like symptoms and little deterioration in personality
Includes the disorders previously termed paranoid psychosis and paraphrenia

F23 Acute and transient psychotic disorders
Mixed group of disorders with an acute onset, which may be stress related, and a brief clinical course
Includes syndromes previously called psychogenic, reactive, and schizophreniform psychoses

F25 Schizoaffective disorders

F30 Manic episode
Hypomania is a mild form without psychotic features

F31 Bipolar affective disorder
Previously termed manic-depressive psychosis
Psychotic symptoms may occur in both manic and depressive phases of illness but are not invariably present

Notes
The disorders listed above are characterised by the presence of psychotic symptoms (delusions and hallucinations). Such symptoms may occur in many mental disorders, including dementias and depression. Schizotypal disorder (F21) is also classified in this group but is regarded by many as primarily a disorder of personality

* World Health Organization. *The ICD-10 classification of mental and behavioural disorders.* Geneva: WHO, 1992

Diagnosis

Presentations evolve over time, from non-specific depression or anxiety into overt psychotic states with typical symptoms. Differential diagnosis is limited, but routine blood tests, a urine screen for drug metabolites, and special investigations are useful to exclude rarer conditions. Temporal lobe epilepsy, cerebral lesions, hypothyroidism (in older patients), and systemic lupus erythematosus are possibilities. The hallucinations associated with alcoholism, illicit drugs, and medications should also be considered.

> **Diagnosis remains a clinical skill, requiring a good social history corroborated by others as well as a detailed assessment of the patient's mental state**

Management

Management requires pharmacological, psychological, and social approaches, depending on the stage of the illness.

Drug treatment

Early treatment with antipsychotic drugs is central to resolving unpleasant symptoms and social impairment. First line treatment requires dopamine blocking drugs such as haloperidol, chlorpromazine, trifluoperazine, sulpiride, and pimozide. Some are available only as oral preparations, and they vary in their sedating and arousing properties as well as side effects.

Continuing treatment—Depot injections giving slow, stable release of drugs over one to four weeks are extremely useful. They enhance compliance, a particular problem in those patients who lack insight. Relief of symptoms is achieved in at least 70% of patients with such treatment.

Advantages of early recognition and treatment

Minimises
- Subjective distress
- Positive symptoms
- Anxiety and depression

Reduces
- Frequency of relapse
- Cognitive deterioration
- Loss of personal self care skills

Limits
- Social disruption and deterioration
- Loss of family support and social networks
- Loss of interpersonal skills

Side effects are a particular problem, especially those affecting movement. Parkinsonian symptoms require antimuscarinic drugs (such as procyclidine or orphenadrine) in a third or more of patients. Sedation or a sense of feeling flattened or depressed may also be distressing. Restlessness, either psychological or affecting the legs (akathisia), is poorly understood but can respond to β blockers. Benzodiazepines usefully treat common problems such as excessive arousal or anxiety or difficulties in sleeping.

Newer "atypical" antipsychotic drugs, such as clozapine or risperidone, have an additional blocking action on serotonin receptors that seems to reduce side effects and negative symptoms. Development of such "cleaner" drugs is one of the most exciting aspects of research in managing schizophrenia.

Psychological treatment

Psychological interventions have centred on work with individual patients to develop social skills. Relapse in schizophrenia seems closely associated with the level of the family's emotional expression as measured by formal assessments of critical comments or expressed hostility in family interviews. Identifying an overinvolved, somewhat angry, and garrulous mother is not difficult.

Fashionable theories of causation in the 1960s, which designated the "schizophrenogenic" parent, have now been discarded. There is, however, a close association between high arousal in the family and early relapse: this can be lowered by structured family education, reducing face-to-face contact via attendance at a day centre, and formal family therapy. Recently, cognitive therapy to reduce the impact of delusional beliefs or hallucinations has shown promise.

Social support

A key worker can help with medication, disability benefits, and housing needs. Hostels or group homes vary in structure and support, from the high dependence units that provide 24 hour care to the semi-independence of a supported flat with someone visiting daily or less often. Day care, whether an active rehabilitation unit aimed at developing job skills or simply support with low key activities, can improve personal functioning (for example hygiene, conversation, and friendships) as well as ensuring early detection of relapse.

There is evidence that targeted community support may reduce the need for respite crisis or compulsory admissions. However, the myth that community care supplants the need for hospital beds is being superseded, particularly where there are high levels of homelessness, such as in the inner cities. A ratio of one acute bed for 10 community placements is probably acceptable.

Prognosis

Prognosis depends on presentation, response to treatment, and the quality of aftercare. Early and continued medication remains the key to good management. Acute onset over several weeks rather than many months, a supportive family, personal intelligence and insight, positive rather than negative symptoms, a later age of onset (over 25 years), and a good response to low doses of drugs are indicative of a better outcome. By contrast, the worst case scenario would be an insidious illness over several years in a teenager from a disrupted family who shows possible brain damage or additional learning difficulties.

What is clear is that the residual population of the old asylums—incontinent, mute, and utterly dependent—is a thing of the past. However, a younger group of constantly

Side effects of antipsychotic drugs

Immediate
- Acute dystonias and dyskinesias
- Sedation
- Dry mouth
- Hypotension
- Akathisia
- Constipation
- Oculogyric crisis
- Neuroleptic malignant syndrome

Medium term (weeks)
- Raised prolactin concentrations, leading to:
  Amenorrhoea
  Subfertility
  Impotence
- Prolonged QTc interval and dysrhythmias
- Weight gain

Long term (months)
- Tardive dyskinesia

> Psychological interventions can minimise distress and reduce frequency of relapse

Psychological and social interventions

With patient
- Training in personal hygiene and self care
- Training in social skills
- Training in budgeting and daily living
- Training in job skills
- Training in anxiety management
- Cognitive therapy for delusions and hallucinations

With patient's family
- Information and support
- Education about illness and its effects
- Telephone helpline for out of hours support
- Self help and carers groups
- Family therapy to reduce high expressed emotion

> Social interventions are the cornerstone of community care

Outcome in schizophrenia

Highly dependent
Up to 20% of sufferers will require long term, highly dependent, structured care, sometimes in locked or secure conditions

Relatively independent
About half of patients can live relatively independent lives, with varying levels of support, but require continuing medication

Independent
The best 30% are independent, working full time, and raising families. Illness with such a good outcome is sometimes termed schizoaffective, and there is continuing debate about the relation between chronic, "process" schizophrenia and those brief psychotic episodes that leave people largely untouched

relapsing patients ("revolving-door patients") shows the limitations of community support. Failure to comply with medication is often a key factor, and research into improving compliance in the community is showing some success.

Outlook

The development of local guidelines and supportive general practices or psychiatric liaison clinics are both educational and effective. Stigma and media hype of isolated assaults (such as the Christopher Clunis affair) tend to mask the good stability and personal functioning of the great majority of patients. Human resources in the form of community psychiatric nurses, social workers, occupational therapists, and care workers are often underestimated as well as underfunded.

Excellent information is obtainable from voluntary groups such as the National Schizophrenia Fellowship or the Hearing Voices Network. New drug and psychological treatments, as well as research insights into the differing syndromes and symptoms, give hope for the future.

Mania and other psychoses

Psychotic symptoms, often indistinguishable from those seen in schizophrenia, occur in manic-depressive illness. Mania typically presents with hyperactivity, an elevated or excessively irritable mood, sleep loss, pressure of speech, and a tendency to jump from topic to topic (flight of ideas). The latter may mimic forms of thought disorder, while grandiose beliefs (often delusional) may generate excess spending or a chaotic personal lifestyle. Hypomania is the term applied to a less severe form without psychotic features.

Modern classification systems recognise the existence of acute and transient psychotic disorders, often occurring in association with stress, which may resolve spontaneously in a few days or weeks. On the other hand, persistent delusional disorder is characterised by circumscribed delusional beliefs of long standing in the absence of other psychotic features or of intellectual deterioration. Schizophrenic or manic symptoms may arise in a range of infective disorders (such as malaria and HIV infection), metabolic disorders (such as hypothyroidism), and idiopathic cerebral disorders.

The artwork is by Melissa Husby and reproduced with permission of the Stock Illustration Source.

> Schizophrenia remains a diagnostic, clinical, and rehabilitative challenge

---

Voluntary organisations

- National Schizophrenia Fellowship (NSF), 28 Castle Street, Kingston upon Thames, Surrey, KT1 1SS
Telephone (0181) 547 3937, Advice Service (0181) 974 6814
Publishes a useful leaflet for patients and families: *What is schizophrenia?* Also a range of leaflets and fact sheets on drug treatments, complementary therapies and claiming benefits (such as Disability Living Allowance).
- Schizophrenia: A National Emergency (SANE), 199-205 Old Marylebone Road, London NW1 5QP
Saneline (0171) 724 8000 and 0345 67 8000
- The Manic Depressive Fellowship has active local groups in many areas
- MIND (National Association for Mental Health), Granta House, 15-17 Broadway, Stratford, London E15 4BQ
Info-Line (0181) 522 1728 and 0345 660 163

Further reading

Barrowclough C, Tarrier N. *Families of schizophrenic patients: cognitive behavioural intervention.* London: Chapman and Hall, 1992

Burns T. Early detection of psychosis in primary care: initial treatment and crisis management. In: Kendrick T, Tylee A, Freeling P, eds. *The prevention of mental illness in primary care.* Cambridge: Cambridge University Press, 1996:246-62

Davies TW. Psychosocial factors and relapse of schizophrenia. *BMJ* 1994;309:353-4.

Long-term management of people with psychotic disorders in the community. *Drug Ther Bull* 1994;32:73-7

Pickar D. Prospects for pharmacotherapy of schizophrenia. *Lancet* 1995;345:557-62

Tylee A. Guidelines for schizophrenia management. *Hospital Update* 1994:(supplement, Psychiatry Seminar):23

Wilkinson G, Kendrick T. *A carer's guide to schizophrenia.* London: Royal Society of Medicine Press, 1996

9   Disorders of personality

Martin Marlowe, Philip Sugarman

Personality disorders are widespread and present a major challenge in most areas of health care. They can be difficult to treat, complicate the management and adversely affect the outcome of other conditions, and exert a disproportionate effect on the workload of staff dealing with them. Finding appropriate placement for sufferers can cause difficulties for doctors and the courts.

Definition and classification

Definition
The study of the personality disorders has been beset by problems, and, as a result, the use of such diagnoses is often questioned. The World Health Organization defines these conditions as comprising "deeply ingrained and enduring behaviour patterns, manifesting themselves as inflexible responses to a broad range of personal and social situations."

They are associated with ways of thinking, perceiving, and responding emotionally that differ substantially from those generally accepted within a patient's culture. As a result, patients tend to exhibit a severely limited repertoire of stereotyped responses in diverse social and personal contexts. These patterns are usually evident during late childhood or adolescence, but the requirement to establish their stability and persistence restricts the use of the term "disorder" to adults.

Classification
There are two main approaches to classification-dimensional and categorical.

Dimensional classification—This defines the degree to which a person displays each of a number of personality traits and behavioural problems. This approach is proving useful in investigating the biochemical underpinnings of many of these disorders.

Categorical classification—This, the basis of the major clinical systems for classifying mental disorders, assumes the existence of distinct types of personality disorder with distinctive features. The World Health Organization's classification of personality disorders has undergone much revision in the past 20 years and has been complicated by the recent addition of behavioural syndromes such as pathological gambling and kleptomania.

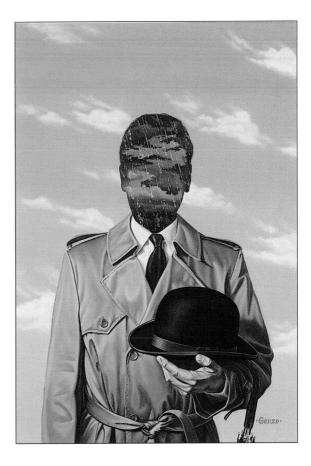

Problems in defining personality disorders

- Confusing terminology derived from different theoretical perspectives
- Two approaches to classification
- Dimensional approach useful in research
- Categorical approach used clinically
- Blurred boundaries with mental illness
- Tendency of clinicians to prefer unitary to multiple diagnoses
- Use of term "personality disorder" as a pejorative label

World Health Organization's classification of personality disorders*

F60-Specific personality disorders
Paranoid—Includes formerly used categories of sensitive and querulant personality
Schizoid—Distinct from schizotypal disorder, which is related to schizophrenia
Dissocial—Formerly called antisocial, asocial, psychopathic, or sociopathic personality
Emotionally unstable—Includes impulsive (explosive) and borderline types
Histrionic—Formerly hysterical personality
Anankastic—Formerly obsessional personality
Anxious—Also called avoidant personality
Dependent—Formerly asthenic, inadequate, or passive personality

F61-Mixed personality disorders
F62-Enduring personality changes
Includes permanent changes after catastrophic experiences (such as hostage taking, torture, or other disaster) or severe mental illness, but excludes changes due to brain damage

F63-Habit and impulse disorders
Includes pathological gambling, fire setting (pyromania), stealing (kleptomania), hair pulling (trichotillomania), and others

F68-Other disorders of personality
A mixed category including elaboration of physical symptoms for psychological reasons and intentional production of symptoms (factitious disorder)

F21 Schizotypal disorder
This category is included for completeness, but it is best avoided as its status as a variant of schizophrenia or of personality disorder is not clear

*ICD-10 (international classification of diseases, 10th edition). This no longer recognises some previously used descriptions of personality disorder as distinct categories. These include eccentric, immature, narcissistic, and passive-aggressive types

---

Epidemiology and aetiology

In Britain the prevalence of personality disorder ranges from 2% to 13% in the general population, and the prevalence is higher in institutional settings (such as in hospitals, residential settings, and prisons). Some diagnoses are made more commonly in men (such as dissocial personality disorder), while others are more common in women (such as histrionic and borderline personality disorders). Some common forms of presentation should prompt consideration of an underlying personality disorder: the association between dissocial personality disorder and alcohol and substance misuse is particularly important.

There are both biological and psychosocial theories of the aetiology of personality and behavioural disorders. Biological and psychosocial theories are not mutually exclusive, and many have contributed to treatment strategies.

Possible causes of personality disorders

- There is mounting evidence to support a genetic component for some behaviours (such as alcoholism of early onset in men)
- Neurochemical research has found serotonin metabolism in the brain to be related to abnormal impulsiveness and aggression
- Some personality disorders can be thought of as attenuated forms of mental illness, the strongest link being between those found in cluster A and schizophrenia
- Psychological theories have focused on failure to progress through early developmental stages as a result of adverse conditions, leading to problems in maintaining relationships in later life

---

Diagnosis of personality disorder

It is generally agreed that the diagnosis of personality disorder of any type should not be made unless certain conditions are met. For practical purposes, these disorders are often grouped into three clusters that share clinical features:

Cluster A—Patients often seem odd or eccentric (such as paranoid or schizoid). Schizotypal disorder is often included in this cluster

Cluster B—Patients may seem dramatic, emotional, or erratic (such as dissocial, histrionic, or borderline type of emotionally unstable personality)

Cluster C—Patients present as anxious or fearful (such as dependent, anxious, anankastic).

Further complications arise because dissocial personality disorder (in the guise of psychopathic disorder or psychopathy) is included in the Mental Health Act 1983 and, if thought to be treatable, can be the basis for compulsory admission to hospital. It is variously defined but can be regarded as a severe example of a cluster B personality disorder.

Prerequisites for diagnosis of personality disorder

Patient displays a pattern of . . .
- Behaviour
- Emotional response
- Perception of self, others and the environment

which is . . .
- Evident in early life
- Persists into adulthood
- Pervasive
- Inflexible
- A deviation from patient's cultural norm

and leads to . . .
- Distress to self, others, or society
- Dysfunction in interpersonal, social, or working relationships

but is not attributable to
- Other psychiatric disorder (such as schizophrenia, depression, drug misuse)
- Other physical disorder (such as acute intoxication, organic brain disease)

Assessment

Patients with personality disorder may present in various ways. Some behaviours suggestive of personality disorder may be overt (such as extreme aggression), but others may be subtle (such as pronounced difficulty in assertiveness or avoidance behaviour). Temporary reactions to particular circumstances do not justify a diagnosis of personality disorder.

Problems presenting for the first time in adulthood may point to a functional or an organic mental illness. A collateral history from a relative or close friend is useful in distinguishing personality traits from mental illness. Patients' social circumstances need to be considered in order to identify solutions to immediate crises. Time spent on the presenting problem may help patients to identify solutions for themselves.

It is important to differentiate personality disorders in cluster A from psychotic mental illness, and personality disorders in cluster C from anxiety and depression whenever possible. However, personality disorder commonly coexists with mental disorder, and a patient may have symptoms of both. Thus, the inclination to withdraw all treatment and support once a personality disorder is suspected should be resisted. Diagnostic uncertainty is an indication for referral to specialist mental health services.

People suffering from personality disorders in cluster B commonly present with aggressive behaviour. Any history of abuse or behavioural disturbance in childhood should be

---

Common presentations of personality disorder

- Aggression
- Alcohol and substance misuse
- Anxiety and depression
- Deliberate self harm
- Bingeing, vomiting, purging, and other eating problems

General practitioners, who may have known a patient since childhood, are in a good position to distinguish between transient and enduring patterns of behaviour

---

Assessment

In addition to routine psychiatric assessment, in cases of suspected personality disorder particular attention should be paid to the following:
- Presenting problems
- Childhood history and experiences, especially of severe illness, abuse or behavioural disturbance
- Reactions to life events
- Violent outbursts or episodes, and their precipitating factors
- Risk taking behaviour
- Relationships, of what kind and how stable
- History of relevant physical disorder, such as head injury, epilepsy, or substance misuse
- Comorbid physical or mental disorders

elicited, and details taken of episodes of violence in public and at home, offending or criminal behaviour, and any experiences of imprisonment. Ideas or threats of harm to self or others should be openly discussed and carefully recorded.

Intervention

The basic principles of intervention include a clear consistent approach, with offers of help being made and delivered within realistic limits. The stance is one of helping patients with their problems without being cast into extreme positions (often as either the "ideal" professional or the "useless" one) or reinforcing avoidance and dependence by denying patients the opportunity to assume responsibility for their actions.

Inevitably, attempting to help a person who has difficulty in forming relationships may be hampered by that difficulty. When several professionals are involved, who is doing what and to what end must be communicated clearly between the professionals and, most importantly, to the patient. Ultimately, developing a working relationship and enhancing the motivation for change are the main foundations of any specific intervention to change behaviour. When these conditions are not met, simple problem solving and recognising and reinforcing individual patients' capacity to change their immediate situation at times of crisis may be useful.

Specific measures
When another disorder coexists the intervention should initially be directed at this but working within the general framework given above. Referral to a specialist service may be indicated for specific problems (such as substance misuse and eating disorder).

Drug treatment—Depot antipsychotic drugs have been reported to benefit patients who harm themselves impulsively, and those who display symptoms suggestive (but falling short) of frank psychotic illness. Serotonin reuptake inhibitors have been used in patients with borderline personality disorder to reported good effect. However, these interventions are not supported by much research evidence, and the benefits of any drug must be weighed against the risk of side effects and toxicity in overdose. Full discussion with individual patients is needed before embarking on such interventions.

Psychosocial intervention—Group and family psychotherapy have their proponents in treating disorders in cluster B on an outpatient basis, but individual cognitive or psychodynamic psychotherapy is usually preferred. Assertiveness training, anxiety management, and behavioural approaches may be useful with disorders in cluster C, as may short term, focused psychotherapy.

Deliberate self harm
There is no clear consensus as to the best management of deliberate self harm in patients with personality disorder. While admission to a general psychiatric hospital may provide apparent safety, security, and containment, self harming may actually worsen—particularly if the admission is unfocused, not part of an overall plan, and the staff have little experience in dealing with the problem.

Aggressive behaviour
In various patient groups aggressive behaviour has been shown to respond to carefully monitored carbamazepine treatment. This is especially true of patients in whom there are associated features such as a history of head injury, genuine amnesia for assaults, the déjà vu phenomenon, olfactory hallucinations, and abnormalities shown by electroencephalography or brain imaging.

General principles of intervention
- Be realistic about what can be delivered, by whom and in what period
- Avoid being cast as angel or tyrant
- Communicate clearly with the patient and other professionals involved
- Aim for a stable, long term therapeutic relationship: this may need to be at a fairly low level of contact
- Aim to improve the patient's
  Self worth
  Problem solving abilities in the short run
  Motivation for change in the long run

Specific measures for intervention
Treat comorbid mental or physical illness
Consider specific drug treatment
- Depot antipsychotic drugs for impulsive self harm
- Selective serotonin reuptake inhibitors for borderline type emotional instability
- Carbamazepine for aggressive behaviour

Consider specific psychological treatments
- Cognitive-behavioural therapy has been found effective in several personality disorders
- Assertiveness training and anxiety management for dependent and anxious patients
- Techniques for managing anger for patients with aggressive behaviour

Self help organisations
- Befriending services or voluntary agencies may support patients with disorders in cluster C and reduce their need for protracted involvement with health services
- Patients with habit disorders can obtain much needed advice and support from self help groups such as Gamblers Anonymous, Narcotics Anonymous, and Alcoholics Anonymous
- Telephone numbers of local and national agencies organising self help groups can be found in the telephone directory or *Yellow Pages*

Managing deliberate self harm
- Admit patients to hospital only as part of a carefully prepared treatment plan
- Relative indications for admission are for assessment of coexisting illness or risk of suicide
- Inpatient contracts, drawn up and signed by patient and staff, have been advocated and may provide a patient with the necessary structure within which help can be offered and received
- The content of a contract must be carefully considered if it is to be a constructive tool rather than a prescription of punishment
- When available, specialist inpatient units allow a much better opportunity for changing recurrent self harm than do general psychiatric units

Psychological techniques for managing anger are useful for patients who are able to tolerate a therapeutic environment and to discuss their own behaviour. The key issue is to identify triggering situations and the automatic patterns of thought that precede an outburst of aggression.

Clinicians who deal with aggressive patients should take basic safety precautions such as not seeing patients in isolated areas and ensuring the availability of alarm systems. More importantly, they should never criticise or admonish such patients and should always try to appear relaxed whatever feelings a patient may engender. Training in break away techniques—physical manoeuvres to escape from an assault—is helpful in maintaining confidence. The boundaries of acceptable and unacceptable behaviour should be clearly explained to patients in the context of helping them to avoid getting into difficulty.

The artwork is by John Paul Genzo and reproduced with permission of the Stock Illustration Source.

Dealing with aggressive patients

- Be supportive to patients—explain their options and choices positively
- Take a forgiving attitude to rudeness
- Don't keep agitated patients waiting
- Don't see patients in isolated areas
- Don't be patronising or tell patients off

Further reading

American Psychiatric Association. *DSM-IV. Diagnostic and statistical manual of mental disorders.* 4th ed. Washington, DC: APA, 1994

Dolan B, Coid J, eds. *Psychopathic and antisocial personality disorders: treatment and research issues.* London: Gaskell, 1993

Tyrer P, Stein G, eds. *Personality disorder reviewed.* London: Gaskell, 1993

World Health Organization. *The ICD-10 classification of mental and behavioural disorders. Clinical descriptions and diagnostic guidelines.* Geneva: WHO, 1992

10 Psychosexual problems

J P Watson, Teifion Davies

Relationship and sexual problems

Sexual problems must be evaluated in terms of the relationships in which they are manifest. Relationships can be classified as stable or unstable and satisfactory or unsatisfactory, and most relationship problems can be thought of as including difficulties with communication, conflict, and commitment. Difficulties tend to vary at different stages of a longstanding relationship such as marriage, accompanying the couple's advancing years. Many sexual problems occur because of threatened or actual rupture of a relationship or separation (including death of a partner).

Close relationships are shaped by the experiences and expectations of the couples and by legal and cultural influences. Three areas commonly require evaluation: implications of unmarried cohabitation rather than marriage, different traditions of relationship of different cultural groups (such as whether marriage partners should be arranged by parents or chosen by the young people), and strong religious beliefs.

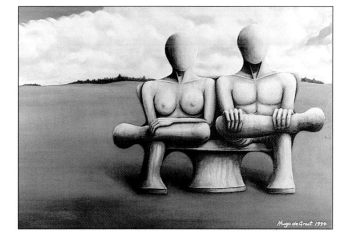

Sexual problems

Four main classes of sexual problems are encountered in clinical practice—sexual dysfunctions (the most common), sexual drive problems, gender problems, and sexual variations and deviations. About 10% of patients attending general practice have some kind of current sexual or relationship difficulty. Three general points are important:
- People vary greatly in the quantity and type of sexual activity they seek to undertake, and in its importance for them
- Whenever a substantial relationship difficulty accompanies sexual dysfunction, one partner is usually the referred patient, but a joint meeting with both partners should be offered. The prognosis is poor if both do not attend for joint meetings
- While it is often easy to identify specifically sexual aspects of a problem, it is difficult to evaluate a couple's relationship from a brief assessment.

Common sexual problems seen in primary care

For practical purposes, the sexual problems seen in primary care may be grouped as
- Sexual dysfunctions
    Primary
    Secondary
- Sexual drive problems
- Gender problems
- Sexual variations and deviations

Classification of adult psychosexual problems★

Behavioural syndromes associated with physiological disturbances and physical factors
F52   Sexual dysfunction not caused by organic disorder or disease
Includes changes in sexual desire or enjoyment, failure of genital response, orgasmic dysfunction, vaginismus, and dyspareunia
Disorders of adult personality and behaviour
F64   Gender identity disorders
Includes transsexualism and disorders in which transvestism occurs but is not accompanied by sexual arousal

F65   Disorders of sexual preference
Includes fetishism, fetishistic transvestism, exhibitionism, voyeurism, paedophilia, sadomasochism, and rarer paraphilias such as those involving animals, rubbing against people in crowds, and making obscene telephone calls
F66   Psychological and behavioural disorders associated with sexual development and orientation
Includes disorders where uncertainty about gender identity or sexual orientation causes distress, or where the individual wishes their gender identity or sexual orientation was different

★ ICD-10 (international classification of diseases, 10th edition). Adult psychosexual problems are classified together with several other types of disorder

---

Sexual dysfunctions

These are problems that make sexual intercourse difficult or impossible. They may be primary (intercourse never adequate) or secondary (intercourse adequate at some time in the past). Erectile and ejaculatory difficulties have similar causes and respond to similar treatments in both heterosexual and homosexual couples.

> **Some degree of sexual dysfunction, most often erection difficulties, occurs at some time during most established relationships**

ABC of mental health

Causes of sexual dysfunction

Efficient sexual function requires anatomical integrity, intact vascular and neurological function, and adequate hormonal control. Peripheral genital efficiency is modulated by excitatory and inhibitory neural connections that mediate psychological influences and which, in turn, are affected by environmental factors.

Sexual dysfunctions are rarely caused by a single factor, although one may predominate. The question is not "Is this problem physical or psychological?" but "How much of each kind of factor operates in this case?" Similar causative factors operate in men and women, but their manifestations are more obvious in men. It is easy to overlook women's problems unless special inquiry is made.

Biological factors

These occur often in the course of chronic physical and mental illnesses. Hypogonadism is a well recognised cause but is not common. Sexual difficulties are rarely due to testosterone deficiency in men or menopausal or menstrual irregularities in women, though the possibility is often entertained, perhaps because doctors are less comfortable evaluating psychological and relationship factors.

It is often the case that no definite biological cause can be found in a particular patient, and other mechanisms are presumed to operate.

Psychological factors

During development, people acquire from their experiences of care givers and others personal models of what people are like. Traumatic experiences with adults during childhood may contribute to later sexual and relationship preferences. However, there is no specific connection between particular experiences of early abuse and later problems, and it is remarkable how often people with awful early experiences emerge relatively intact. Nevertheless, the responses of an adult to a prospective sexual partner are framed by expectations of how "a person like that" will behave.

Cognitions (thoughts) and moods (emotions) shape each person's experience of sexual arousal and behaviour. Attentional processes are important: in the common experience of spectatoring, people focus on their own performance, often expecting failure, rather than on the sensuality of lovemaking. Pain, ruminations, and worries divert attention.

Intense negative emotions tend to reduce sexual activity and performance, but the association is not close. In depression, sexual enjoyment is often diminished but occasionally increased; the preferred erotic behaviour may alter, often becoming more passive; and antidepressant drugs may adversely affect sexual response.

Environmental factors

Inanimate and animate aspects of the environment profoundly affect sexual arousal and response and, of course, determine whether intimate behaviour will take place at all, as well as its efficiency and enjoyability. This includes where and when sex takes place, the ambient temperature, who else is present or nearby, light or darkness, clothing, and so forth. Whether particular circumstances are excitatory or inhibitory is largely culturally determined.

Assessing sexual dysfunction

The affected behaviours should be elicited in detail—who is doing what, to whom, and in what circumstances?

The onset of a problem should be specified. A gradual onset, especially after previously satisfactory sexual activity and with

Common sexual dysfunctions

Men
- Erectile impotence (loss of penile rigidity sufficient to allow efficient coitus)
- Premature ejaculation (ejaculation occurring sooner than is wished)

Women
- Failure to arouse or to achieve orgasm
- Vaginismus (involuntary spasmodic problem in pelvic floor muscles making penetration difficult or impossible)

Common biological causes of sexual dysfunction
- Neuropathy (arteriopathy is less common)
- Hypertension
- Ischaemic vascular disease
- Side effects of drugs used to treat diabetes or hypertension
- Other drugs including antidepressants
- Alcohol

Chronic illnesses causing sexual dysfunction
- Diabetes
- Multiple sclerosis
- Cerebrovascular accidents
- Post-traumatic states including paraplegia
- Schizophrenia
- Depression
- Manic-depressive disorder

Some important psychological factors in sexual dysfunction
- Previous experience
- Expectation (of failure)
- Attention
- Anxiety
- Worries and ruminations
- Depression
- Pain

Genital responsiveness is the final common path issuing from many interacting influences: biological, psychological, and social

a good concurrent relationship, points to an important physical cause. However, it is often impossible to identify what physical factors are involved. The timing and circumstances of altered sexual interest, and its association with interpersonal conflicts should be noted.

Psychological causes of sexual dysfunctions should be identified positively and not merely by exclusion. Common attributional biases may cloud the issue: women tend to blame themselves for marital difficulties and the sexual complaints of their partners, or to blame their menstrual (or menopausal) status for loss of sexual interest or other difficulties. Both men and women find it easier to blame medication for sexual problems than the much more common conflicts in a relationship or family.

A physical examination is an essential part of the assessment, but the doctor should be sensitive to its potential emotional impact. It is usually best for women patients with sexual complaints to be examined by women.

Investigating sexual dysfunction

Appropriate investigations will depend on the patient's history, and specialist referral may also be considered. If the referrer is almost certain that an important physical factor is relevant, referral to a specialist urological or medical clinic may be made. However, when there is any suggestion that psychological factors are involved, then referral to a sexual and relationships clinic, if available, is likely to provide a more comprehensive service.

In cases of erectile failure, intracavernosal injection of papaverine or prostaglandin E1 may be useful initially as an investigation under carefully controlled conditions, and both these drugs can become treatments. Patients with diabetic neuropathy usually respond well to injection, while those with arteriopathic conditions do not.

Treating sexual dysfunction

Treatment involves attention to physical, psychological, and social aspects: all should be considered in every case.

Physical treatments

An exclusively biological approach without full conversational inquiry is not satisfactory and increases the chance of treatment failure or relapse. Nevertheless, the treatment of impotence has been revolutionised in recent years by the development of improved physical methods, including intracavernosal injections; the use of a vacuum device; various creams and ointments containing nitrite, which may be beneficial when rubbed into the penis; and the operative insertion of semi-rigid rods, which may provide a semi-erection sufficient for coitus.

Psychosocial treatments

These include general counselling to allow attentive exploration of concerns and specific counselling for the cognitive distortions that may accompany mood problems. Some techniques are derived from the "Masters and Johnson" approach, which includes non-genital intimacy during an agreed ban on sexual intercourse to alleviate anxiety about performance and a "stop-start" approach to improve ejaculatory control. Treatment goals should be agreed, which can be approached gradually so as to replace experiences of failure with successes and anxiety with enjoyment. This usually entails practice ("homework") between sessions.

Specific couple therapy may be necessary to treat problems with communication or to enhance a couple's skills in resolving conflict and solving problems. These methods are well suited for use in primary care.

Example of a case history

A businessman aged 50 consulted for gradually worsening impotence of three years' duration. His business had failed four years previously, and his wife had divorced him six months later. Three years ago a routine medical examination had disclosed important hypertension, for which a β blocker had been prescribed, and he had been advised to reduce his alcohol intake from his habitual 30 units a week.

This not uncommon type of history mentions five factors plausibly related to erectile difficulty: work and marital stress (psychological factors) and hypertension, drug treatment, and alcohol (physical factors)

Help with sexual problems

Sexual and relationships clinics
A list of clinics is available from
   The Honorary Secretary, British Association of   Sexual and Marital Therapy, PO Box 62, Sheffield   S10 3TS

Brook Advisory Centres
Adolescents and young adults may find the advice and counselling on sexual problems offered by Brook Advisory Centres to be particularly welcome. Telephone numbers of local centres are available from (0171) 713 9000

Leaflet
Depression and your sex life by Dr David Baldwin. Available from: Depression Alliance, PO Box 1022, London SE1 7QB (Answerphone (0171) 721 7672)

Many men are given androgen preparations after consultations about impotence. This is useless in the absence of androgen deficiency with signs of hypogonadism in addition to sexual changes

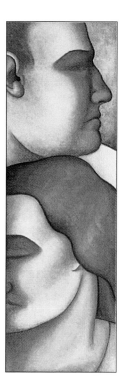

Sexual drive problems

Men and women often have feelings of inferiority about their sexual capacity, but this is not an illness. Loss of (or, less commonly, increase in) sexual drive or interest is common in both men and women. This may manifest in changes in thoughts, fantasies, experienced urges, inclination to initiate sexual activity, or specific changes in sexual behaviour. The term "libido" is vague and best avoided.

Gender problems

Serious problems of gender may accompany endocrinological and developmental disorders that produce ambiguous external genitalia or excessive masculinisation or feminisation.

Transsexualism is a gender identity disorder characterised by a lifelong feeling that your true gender is discordant from your phenotype. This is associated with an insistent search for gender reassignment procedures, most notably for surgical intervention to make the body more concordant with the experienced self. It affects about one in 700 people and is 10 times more common in men than women. In adults the treatment is to use social, medical, and surgical measures to help patients achieve their aims, rather than to try to alter their gender identity. Surgical procedures remain controversial but can produce considerable psychological benefit in selected cases.

Sexual variations and deviations

The paraphilias are problems arising from sexual preferences that are unwelcome to the patients, to others, or to society at large. They represent modifications of the capacity for erotic response to another adult and can be understood as a disconnection between sex and affection. Most paraphilias involve behaviours that play a small part in usual adult lovemaking—for example, exposing, sexual looking, dominating, submitting, dressing up, and regard for particular objects. In a paraphilia, however, such behaviour becomes the erotic end in itself.

While a wide range of paraphiliac activities has been described, recurring patterns include sadomasochism (the infliction or experience of pain), transvestism (cross dressing), fetishism, and various illegal activities such as exposing the genitals in public and sexual preference for prepubertal children. The assessment and treatment of paraphilias is a specialist matter. Psychological treatments are often of considerable value, but the availability of services is very patchy and awareness of local arrangements is essential.

Gender identity is a person's sense that he or she is male, female, or ambivalent. Core gender identity is established by the age of 4 or 5 years
Gender role is the public expression of a person's gender

Paraphilias may occur in people given to heterosexual, homosexual, or bisexual preferences. Homosexual preference is not a problem in itself and is best regarded as a status (like left handedness)

Further reading

Dawson C, Whitfield H. *ABC of urology.* London: BMJ Publishing Group, 1996

Gregoire A, Pryor JP. *Impotence: an integrated approach to clinical practice.* Edinburgh: Churchill Livingstone, 1993

Spence SH. *Psychosexual therapy. A cognitive-behavioural approach.* London: Chapman and Hall, 1991

Wellings K, Field J, Johnson AM, Wadsworth J. *Sexual behaviour in Britain. The national survey of sexual attitudes and lifestyles.* London: Penguin Books, 1994

The artwork on page 35 is by Hugo deGroot and on the third page by Sandra Dionisi; they are reproduced with permission of the Stock Illustration Source.

11 Addiction and dependence—Illicit drugs

Claire Gerada, Mark Ashworth

Size of the problem

About 30% of adults in Britain have used illicit drugs at some time in their lives, but misuse of prescription drugs (such as benzodiazepines and barbiturates) is probably even more widespread. Cannabis is the most commonly used illicit drug. About 100 000 people misuse heroin (diamorphine), and an unknown but increasing number use other drugs such as ecstasy and amphetamines.

While the number of new drug users continues to rise (Fig 11.1), the number who inject drugs is falling, possibly as a result of health education about risks of HIV transmission. The highest number of addicts are found in London and the north west of England.

Why misuse drugs?

What determines whether drug use becomes continuous and problematic includes (Fig 11.2)
- Sociocultural factors such as cost and availability of the drug
- Controls and sanctions on its use
- Age (people in their teens to their 20s are most at risk) and sex (male)
- Peer group of the person taking the drug.

Personality factors determine how a person copes once addicted and the mechanisms he or she may use to seek help.

Commonly misused drugs

Common drugs of misuse tend to cause dependence and euphoria.

Benzodiazepines

This is the largest category of drug misuse. The most commonly misused drugs, temazepam and diazepam, usually originate from legal prescriptions or thefts from pharmacies. They may be taken alone as the drug of choice, to supplement opioids, or as a last resort when supply of opioids fails. Tolerance to benzodiazepines can occur, with daily doses escalating to 50-100 mg of diazepam. Intravenous injection of the viscous gel within temazepam capsules can cause catastrophic embolic damage to limbs and digits: temazepam is now a controlled drug.

A withdrawal syndrome can occur after only three weeks of continuous use, and it affects a third of long term users. The syndrome usually consists of increased anxiety and perceptual disturbances, especially heightened sensitivity to light and sound; occasionally there are fits, hallucinations, and confusion. Depending on the drug's half life, symptoms start one to five days after the last dose, peak within 10 days, and subside after one to six weeks.

Opioids

Opioids produce an intense but transient feeling of pleasure. Withdrawal symptoms begin a few hours from the last dose, peak after two to three days, and subside after a week. Heroin (diamorphine) is available in a powdered form, commonly mixed ("cut") with other substances such as chalk or lactose

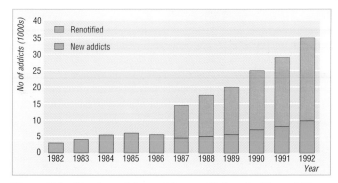

Figure 11.1   Numbers of drug addicts notified to the Home Office during 1982–92

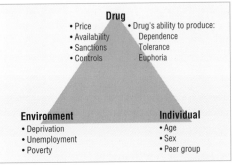

Figure 11.2   Factors influencing misuse of drugs

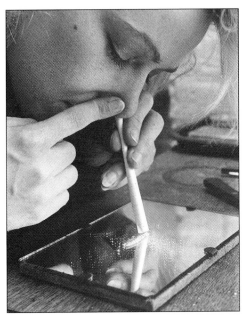

Figure 11.3   Snorting heroin (picture reproduced with subject's permission)

Heroin withdrawal syndrome
- Insomnia
- Muscle pains and cramps
- Increased salivary, nasal, and lacrimal secretions
- Anorexia, nausea, vomiting, and diarrhoea
- Dilated pupils
- Yawning

powder. It can be sniffed ("snorting" (Fig 11.3)), eaten, smoked ("chasing the dragon" (Fig 11.4)), injected subcutaneously ("skin popping"), or injected intravenously ("mainlining"). Tablets can be crushed and then injected.

Amphetamines

These cause generalised overarousal with hyperactivity, tachycardia, dilated pupils, and fine tremor. These effects last about three to four hours, after which the user becomes tired, anxious, irritable, and restless. High doses and chronic use can produce psychosis with paranoid delusions, hallucinations, and overactivity. Physical dependence can occur, and termination of prolonged use may cause profound depression and lassitude. Amphetamines were widely prescribed in the 1960s: the most common current source is illegally produced amphetamine sulphate powder, which can be taken by mouth, by sniffing, or by intravenous injection.

Cocaine

Cocaine preparations can be eaten (coca leaves or paste), injected alone or with heroin ("speedballing"), sniffed ("snow"), or smoked (as "crack"). Crack is cocaine in its base form and is smoked because of the speed and intensity of its psychoactive effects. The stimulant effect ("rush") is felt within seconds of smoking crack, peaks in one to five minutes, and wears off after about 15 minutes.

Smokable cocaine produces physical dependence with craving: the withdrawal state is characterised by depression and lethargy followed by increased craving, which can last up to three months. Overdose by any route can result in death from myocardial infarction, hyperthermia, or ventricular arrhythmias.

Ecstasy (3,4-methylenedioxymethamphetamine, MDMA)

An increasingly popular drug, especially at "rave" parties, ecstasy (known as "E") has hallucinogenic properties and produces euphoria and increased energy. Continuous or excessive use with raised physical activity can lead to death through hyperthermia and dehydration.

Misused volatile substances

Such substances include glues (the most common), gas fuels, cleaning agents, correcting fluid thinners, and aerosols. Their main misuse is among young boys as part of a group activity; those who misuse alone tend to be more disturbed and in need of psychiatric help. Their effects are similar to alcohol: intoxication with initial euphoria followed by disorientation, blurred vision, dizziness, slurred speech, ataxia, and drowsiness. About 100 people die each year from misusing volatile substances, mainly from direct toxic effects.

Dependence syndrome

The dependence syndrome is a cluster of symptoms, not all of which need be present for a diagnosis of dependence to be made. The key feature is a compulsion to use drugs, which results in overwhelming priority being given to drug-seeking behaviour. Other features are tolerance (need to increase drug dose to achieve desired effect), withdrawal (both physical and psychological symptoms on stopping use), and use of drug to relieve or avoid withdrawal symptoms. An addict's increasing focus on drug-seeking behaviour leads to progressive loss of other interests, neglect of self care and social relationships, and disregard for harmful consequences.

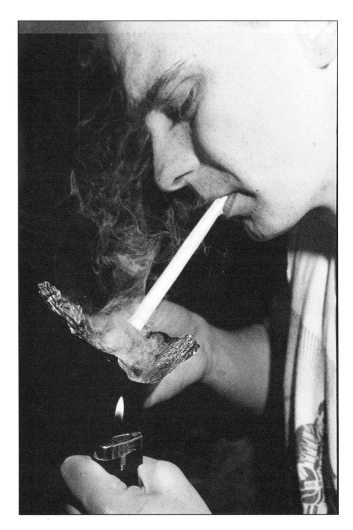

Figure 11.4 "Chasing the dragon"—smoking heroin (picture reproduced with subject's permission)

Clinical conditions associated with drug misuse

Several clinical conditions are recognised as arising from misuse of drugs. Their clinical features are similar regardless of the drug misused:

Acute intoxication—May be uncomplicated or associated with bodily injury, delirium, convulsions, or coma. Includes "bad trips" due to hallucinogenic drugs

Harmful use—A pattern of drug misuse resulting in physical harm (such as hepatitis) or mental harm (such as depression) to the user. These consequences often elicit negative reactions from other people and result in social disruption for the user

Dependence syndrome—Obtaining and using the drug assume the highest priorities in the user's life. A person may be dependent on a single substance (such as diazepam), a group of related drugs (such as the opioids), or a wide range of different drugs. This is the state known colloquially as drug addiction

Withdrawal—Usually occurs when a patient is abstinent after a prolonged period of drug use, especially if large doses were used. Withdrawal is time limited, but withdrawal may cause convulsions and require medical treatment

Psychotic disorder—Any drug can produce the hallucinations, delusions, and behavioural disturbances characteristic of psychosis. Patterns of symptoms may be extremely variable, even during a single episode. Early onset syndromes (within 48 hours) may mimic schizophrenia or psychotic depression; late onset syndromes (after two weeks or more) include flashbacks, personality changes, and cognitive deterioration

Medical complications of drug misuse

Complications can arise secondary to the drug used (such as constipation), route of drug use (such as deep vein thrombosis), and the lifestyle associated with a drug habit (such as crime). Complications commonly arise from injecting drugs: using dirty and non-sterile needles risks cellulitis, endocarditis, and septicaemia; sharing injecting equipment ("works") can transmit HIV, hepatitis B, and hepatitis C; and incorrect technique can result in venous thrombosis or accidental arterial puncture.

A major hazard of intravenous misuse is overdose, which may be accidental or deliberate. Death from intravenous opioid overdose can be rapid. Opioid overdose should be suspected in any unconscious patient, especially in combination with pinpoint pupils and respiratory depression. Immediate injection of the opioid antagonist naloxone can be lifesaving.

Practical management

General principles
- Prevent misuse by careful prescribing of potential drugs of misuse such as analgesics, hypnotics, and tranquillisers
- Encourage patients into treatment
- Reduce harm associated with drug use
- Treat physical complications of drug use and interactions with prescribed drugs
- Offer general medical care (such as hepatitis immunisation and cervical screening)
- Refer to specialist treatment centre (such as Council for Involuntary Addiction or Narcotics Anonymous). As well as statutory services, many local voluntary and self help groups such as Narcotics Anonymous and Turning Point can provide much needed advice and support for patients with drug related problems. Most voluntary agencies prefer patients to make contact directly. Details may be found in the telephone directory or *Yellow Pages*, or obtained from:
- Standing Conference on Drug Abuse (SCODA), Waterbridge House, 32 Loman Street, London WC1 0EE.

Specific measures
The full drug history must include substances taken, duration and frequency of use, amount of drug used (recorded verbatim), and route of drug use. It is useful to ask the cost of the patient's daily habit as confirmation of use—1 g of street heroin costs £80–£100; users' average daily use is up to 1 g heroin a day.

Injecting users will have needle track marks, usually in the antecubital fossae, although any venous site can be used. Further investigation should include a (fresh) urine drug screen and contacting the NHS regional database to confirm a user's history of treatment and to establish whether the person is already in receipt of a prescription.

Withdrawal from non-opioid drugs
To withdraw a patient from any benzodiazepine, first convert the misused drug into an equivalent dose of diazepam, which has a long half life. Reduce the diazepam dose by 2 mg a fortnight over a period of two to six months. Do not use other drugs to aid withdrawal without a specific indication (such as antidepressants, buspirone, β blockers, carbamazepine).

There is no recommended substitution treatment for cocaine or amphetamines, and they may be withdrawn abruptly. Antidepressants in therapeutic doses may help specific symptoms. Cannabis, ecstasy, and volatile (solvent) substances may all be withdrawn abruptly, but abstinence is more likely to be maintained if attention is paid to any psychological symptoms that emerge.

Complications of injecting drug use

Poor injecting technique
- Abscess
- Cellulitis
- Thrombophlebitis
- Arterial puncture
- Deep vein thrombosis

Needle sharing
- Hepatitis B and C
- HIV or AIDS

Drug content or contaminants
- Abscess
- Overdose
- Gangrene
- Thrombosis

Important interactions between illicit and prescribed drugs

Amphetamines
Chlorpromazine—Antipsychotic effects opposed
Lithium carbonate—No harmful effects reported. Reduces the "high"
Monoamine oxidase inhibitors—Potentially fatal hypertensive crisis

Cannabis
Fluoxetine—Increased energy, hypersexuality, pressured speech
Tricyclic antidepressants—Marked tachycardia

Cocaine
Monoamine oxidase inhibitors—Possibility of hypertension

Ecstasy
Phenelzine—Hypertension

Opioids
Desipramine—Methadone doubles serum levels of desipramine
Diazepam—Increased central nervous system depression
Monoamine oxidase inhibitors—Potentially fatal interaction with pethidine

Data from Neil Spencer, principal pharmacist, Lambeth Healthcare NHS Trust

---

Useful contacts and telephone numbers

- British Doctors' and Dentists' Group. (Independent professional self help organisation for alcohol and drug dependent doctors and dentists). (0171)487 4445/(01252) 316776
- Council for Involuntary Addiction (CITA) (0151) 949 0102
- Narcotics Anonymous (0171) 351 6794
- Turning Point (0171) 702 2300
- *D-mag* is an informative magazine for young people published by the Institute for the Study of Drug Dependence and the Health Education Authority. For copies, telephone the National Drugs Helpline on 0800 776600. Advice is available in several languages

---

Factors to be recorded in a drug assessment

Drug taken
- Opioids—Heroin, methadone, buprenorphine (Temgesic), dihydrocodeine (DF 118), others
- Benzodiazepines
- Stimulants—Cocaine, amphetamines, ecstasy, others
- Alcohol

Amount taken
In weight (g), cost (£), volume (ml), No of tablets

Route of administration
Intravenous, intramuscular, subcutaneous, oral, inhaled

Benzodiazepines in equivalent doses of diazepam

Diazepam 10 mg is approximately equivalent to

- Alprazolam (Xanax)	1 mg
- Chlordiazepoxide (Librium, Tropium)	30 mg
- Flunitrazepam (Rohypnol)	2 mg
- Flurazepam (Dalmane)	30 mg
- Loprazolam (Dormonoct)	1 mg
- Lorazepam (Ativan)	1 mg
- Lormetazepam	1 mg
- Nitrazepam (Mogadon, Remnos)	10 mg
- Oxazepam	30 mg
- Temazepam (Normison)	20 mg

Data from sources including *British National Formulary* and *Monthly Index of Medical Specialties (MIMS)*

Treating opioid dependence

Do not start methadone treatment for patients with small habits (less than 0·25 g heroin a day) or where follow up is difficult (such as a patient seen in an accident and emergency department). Propranolol and co-phenotrope (Lomotil) provide symptomatic relief from opioid withdrawal in these patients. Expect only limited enthusiasm with the offer of this treatment.

For patients with more severe physical dependence or pregnant heroin users, for whom acute withdrawal can precipitate premature labour, methadone mixture 1 mg/ml is indicated. Any doctor can prescribe methadone. It is an effective long acting opioid substitute, unlikely to be injected, and with a low resale value on the black market. With the linctus formulation it is very difficult to obtain a "high" so death can arise from inadvertent overdose as naïve users increase the dose expecting euphoric effects.

To assess the required dose: firstly, either calculate the approximate methadone dose or prescribe 10-30 mg methadone a day; and, secondly, assess daily for withdrawal symptoms for a few days, increasing by small increments (such as 5-10 mg) until the patient is comfortable.

Irrespective of their alleged heroin use most patients can be stabilised on 40-60 mg methadone a day, and no more than 60 mg a day should be prescribed without the help of a specialist agency. After a period of stabilisation, reductions in dose should be negotiated with patients and can be 5 mg per week or per fortnight. An agreed treatment plan, allowing some flexibility, should be adhered to as patients benefit from the stability that a methadone prescription brings to their lives.

How to prescribe opioids

General practitioners can use blue FP10 (MDA) prescriptions, which allow daily instalments on a single prescription, thus reducing the risk of overdose or diversion into the black market.

Prescriptions for controlled drugs must:

- Be written in indelible ink
- Be signed and dated by the doctor
- State the form and strength of the preparation
- State doses in words and figures
- State the total dose
- Specify the amount in each instalment and the intervals between instalments.

Opioids in equivalent doses of methadone

Drug	Dose	Methadone equivalent
Dipipanone (Diconal)	10 mg tablet	4 mg
Dihydrocodeine (DF 118)	30 mg tablet	3 mg
Dextromoramide (Palfium)	5 mg tablet	5-10 mg
	10 mg tablet	10-20 mg
Buprenorphine (Temgesic)	200 µg tablet	5 mg
	300 µg ampoule	8 mg
Pentazocine (Fortral)	50 mg capsule	4 mg
	25 mg tablet	2 mg
Codeine Linctus 100 ml	300 mg codeine phosphate	10 mg
Codeine phosphate	15 mg tablet	1 mg
	30 mg tablet	2 mg
	60 mg tablet	3 mg
Street heroin	Cannot be estimated accurately because street drugs vary in purity. Titrate dose against withdrawal symptoms: 1 g heroin = about 40-60 ml methadone	
Pharmaceutical heroin	10 mg tablet or ampoule	20 mg
	30 mg ampoule	50 mg
Pharmaceutical methadone (Physeptone)	10 mg/ml ampoule	10 mg
	Mixture (1 mg/ml) 10 ml	10 mg
	Linctus (2 mg/5 ml) 10 ml	4 mg
	5 mg tablets	5 mg
Street methadone	May have been watered down: titrate dose against withdrawal symptoms	
Pethidine	50 mg tablet 50 mg ampoule	5 mg 5 mg
Morphine	10 mg ampoule	10 mg

Adapted from: *Drug misuse and dependence. Guidelines on clinical management.* London: HMSO, 1991

Notification

On 1 May 1997 the Home Office Addicts Index, which removed the statutory obligation on doctors to report addicts to the Home Office, was discontinued. It remains good practice, however, for doctors to complete the relevant NHS regional database which has now become the only national ongoing source of statistical information regarding drug users contacting doctors. This database holds only basic patient details (initials, birth date and sex) and therefore has a limited use in providing information about patients' contact with other members of the medical profession.

> **Health authorities will be able to put doctors in touch with their regional database. As yet there is no central telephone number**

Further reading

Chick J, Cantwell R, eds. *Seminars in alcohol and drug abuse.* London: Gaskell, 1994

Department of Health. *Drug misuse and dependence. Guidelines on clinical management.* London: HMSO, 1991

Farrell M, Gerada C. Drug misusers: Whose business is it? *BMJ* 1997; 315: 559–60

Helping patients who misuse drugs. *Drug Ther Bull* 1997;35:18–22

Russell J, Lader M, eds. *Guidelines for the prevention and treatment of benzodiazepine dependence.* London: Mental Health Foundation, 1993

Williams H, Ghodse H. The prevention of alcohol and drug misuse. In: Kendrick T, Tylee A, Freeling P, eds. *The prevention of mental illness in primary care.* Cambridge: Cambridge University Press, 1996:223–45

Williams H, Salter M, Ghodse AH. Management of substance misusers on the general hospital ward. *Br J Clin Pract* 1996;50:94–8

The photographs of drug users are by and reproduced with permission of David Hoffman.

12 Addiction and dependence—Alcohol

Mark Ashworth, Claire Gerada

Prevalence of alcohol related problems

As with any drug of addiction, there are four levels of alcohol use.

Social drinking—Only about 10% of the population are teetotal.

At risk consumption—This is the level of alcohol intake that, if maintained, poses a risk to health. *The Health of the Nation* gives "safe" levels of consumption—21 units a week for men and 14 units for women. These levels are exceeded by a sizeable minority of the population—28% of men and 11% of women.

Problem drinking—At this level, consumption causes serious problems to drinkers, their family and social network, or to society. About 1-2% of the population have alcohol problems.

Dependence and addiction—The characteristics of dependence apply to alcohol as to other drugs—periodic or chronic intoxication, uncontrollable craving, tolerance resulting in dose increase, dependence (either psychological or physical), and a detrimental result to the person or society. There are about 200 000 dependent drinkers in the United Kingdom.

Factors aecting consumption

Consumption of alcohol depends on several variables.

Sex—Although men are twice as likely to have alcohol related problems, the gap between the sexes is narrowing.

Occupation—Alcohol misuse is more common in jobs related to catering, brewing, and distilling. In others, such as doctors, sailors, and demolition workers, high consumption is perceived as the social norm.

Homelessness—About a third of homeless people have alcohol problems.

Race—British Afro-Caribbeans and south Asians have lower average consumption and lower hospital admission rates for alcohol related problems than white people. However, pockets of high consumption exist, as has been reported among Sikh men (particularly of spirits). About a fifth of Chinese and Japanese people cannot drink alcohol because of an inherited lack of the liver enzyme acetaldehyde dehydrogenase.

Recognising problem drinking

Recognising people with alcohol related problems is difficult—probably less than 20% are known to their general practitioner, and a large proportion are missed in accident and emergency departments. Recognition is particularly difficult among teenagers, elderly people, and doctors. About half of the doctors reported to the General Medical Council for health difficulties liable to affect professional competence have an alcohol problem.

Doctors may be alerted to an alcohol problem by the presenting complaint. The essential first stage in improving recognition is taking a drinking history, and this should be combined with selected investigations.
- Amount of alcohol consumed in units. Always inquire about quantity and type of drink. Many doctors are unaware of the unit values for common descriptions of daily intake
- Time of first alcoholic drink of the day
- Pattern of drinking: problem drinking is characterised by the establishment of an unvarying pattern of daily drinking

---

> Alcohol exacts a huge toll on the nation's physical, social, and psychological health. Consumption doubled between 1950 and 1980, during which time the relative price of alcohol halved. Since then consumption has flattened off

---

Alcohol related problems
- 33 000 premature deaths a year in England and Wales are related to alcohol consumption
- 300 of these deaths are the direct result of alcoholic liver damage (the true figure is probably many times higher but is hidden by underreporting on death certificates)

Alcohol consumption is associated with
- 80% of suicides
- 50% of murders
- 80% of deaths from fire
- 40% of road traffic accidents
- 30% of fatal road traffic accidents
- 15% of drownings

Alcohol consumption contributes to
- 1 in 3 divorces
- 1 in 3 cases of child abuse
- 20-30% of all hospital admissions

> People lacking the liver enzyme acetaldehyde dehydrogenase experience extremely unpleasant reactions on exposure to alcohol because of accumulation of acetaldehyde. Reactions include nausea, flushing, headache, palpitations and collapse.
> Alcohol evokes a similar response in patients who are given disulfiram

---

Alcohol content of alcoholic drinks
1 unit of alcohol = 1 cl alcohol = about 10 g

Beers, lagers, cider
1 pint = 2 units
1 can = $1\frac{1}{2}$ units

Low alcohol beers, lagers, cider
1 pint = $\frac{2}{3}$ unit
1 can = $\frac{1}{2}$ unit

Strong beers, lagers, cider
1 pint = 3 units
1 can = $2\frac{1}{4}$ units

Extra strong beers, lagers, cider
1 pint = 5 units
1 can = 4 units

Table wine
1 glass = 1 unit
1 bottle (75 cl) = 8 units

Sherry
1 standard small measure = 1 unit
1 bottle = 13 units

Spirits
1 standard measure (England and Wales) = 1 unit
1 standard measure (Scotland and Northern Ireland) = $1\frac{1}{2}$ units
1 bottle = 30 units

Be on your guard for
- "Alco-pops"—These are increasingly popular mixtures of alcohol and fruit flavoured drink. One bottle contains $1\frac{1}{2}$ units of alcohol (equivalent to a can of lager)
- Extra strong lager is relatively cheap but contains 4 units of alcohol per can (equivalent to two pints of ordinary beer)

- Presence of withdrawal symptoms such as early morning shakes or nausea.

Specific questioning should continue with the CAGE questionnaire. Investigation should include measuring the mean corpuscular volume and γ-glutamyl transferase activity. This combination of tests will detect about 75% of people with an alcohol problem, while measuring γ-glutamyl transferase alone detects only a third of cases.

<table>
<tr><td>

CAGE questionnaire[1]

Alcohol dependence is likely if the patient gives two or more positive answers to the following questions:
- Have you ever felt you should **C**ut down on your drinking?
- Have people **A**nnoyed you by criticising your drinking?
- Have you ever felt bad or **G**uilty about your drinking?
- Have you ever had a drink first thing in the morning to steady your nerves or get rid of a hangover (**E**ye-opener)?

[1] Ewing JA. Detecting alcoholism—the CAGE questionnaire. *JAMA* 1984; **252**: 1905–7.

</td></tr>
</table>

Presentation of alcohol problems or dependence

Social presentations

Probably the most common presentations, they include
- Requests for medical certificates
- Marital problems, divorce, domestic violence
- Financial problems, absenteeism, accidents at work
- Public drunkenness or aggression, football hooliganism
- Prosecutions for violent behaviour or driving offences, sexual assault, and vagrancy

Medical presentations

About 80% of patients referred for treatment of alcohol misuse have important medical problems. Withdrawal symptoms are often experienced on waking. Features of specific complications are extremely varied:
Gastrointestinal—hepatitis, cirrhosis, gastritis, gastrointestinal haemorrhage, pancreatitis
Cardiovascular—hypertension (causing increased rates of cerebrovascular and coronary artery disease), arrhythmias, cardiomyopathy
Cancers—mouth, oesophagus, liver, and possibly colon and breast
Obstetric—fetal alcohol syndrome
Neurological—blackouts, fits, neuropathy, acute confusional states, subdural haematoma, Wernicke's encephalopathy, Korsakoff's psychosis
Musculoskeletal—gout

Psychiatric presentations

Depression—All the features of depression can be induced by alcohol. Depression can itself cause alcoholism by triggering drinking in an attempt to relieve some of the depressive symptoms
Anxiety—These symptoms often present during partial withdrawal. Just as with depression, an anxiety or panic disorder can predispose to alcohol excess in an attempt to relieve symptoms
Personality change—Decline in the usual standards of social concern and personal care
Sexual dysfunction—Impotence, delayed ejaculation
Hallucinations—Both auditory and visual, usually during withdrawal but can occur without the other features of delirium tremens
Alcoholic hallucinosis—Rare, distressing auditory hallucinations occurring in clear consciousness

Managing problem drinking

Brief intervention

Randomised controlled trials have shown general practitioners' interventions to be effective. Brief intervention consists of assessing the patient's alcohol intake, providing information about the effects of alcohol, giving advice on reducing consumption, and "motivational interviewing." Although simple, this form of intervention achieves more than a 20% reduction in alcohol consumption among problem drinkers.

Other specialist options, such as inpatient or outpatient care and long term counselling, are available, but there is little evidence that any of these are more effective than brief intervention.

Controlled drinking or abstinence

If drinking is excessive but largely without problems then controlled drinking can be a realistic option. Tactics to achieve this include reducing the alcoholic strength of drinks, spacing drinks, alternating alcoholic with non-alcoholic drinks, and eating with drinks.

Abstinence is recommended if there is established alcohol dependence, marked physical damage, or when controlled drinking has failed. Abstinence should be long term, but some patients succeed in returning to controlled drinking after a period of abstinence. An unrealistic emphasis on abstinence may be counterproductive and end up triggering spectacular relapse.

Managing alcohol dependence

Detoxification

Alcohol dependence usually requires controlled detoxification with an attenuation therapy (such as a benzodiazepine) since abrupt cessation of alcohol can induce one of the withdrawal states. Detoxification is increasingly taking place in the

> About a third of people who seriously misuse alcohol recover without any professional intervention

Classification of alcohol related disorders

Acute intoxication—At low doses, alcohol may have stimulant effects, but these give way to agitation and, ultimately, sedation at higher doses. "Drunkenness" may be uncomplicated or may lead to hangover, trauma, delirium, convulsions, or coma
Pathological intoxication—A state in which even small quantities of alcohol produce sudden, uncharacteristic outbursts of violent behaviour
Harmful use—Actual physical or mental harm to the user, and associated disruption of his or her social life
Dependence syndrome—Craving for alcohol that overrides the normal social constraints on drinking. This state is known colloquially as alcoholism and includes dipsomania
Withdrawal states—With or without delirium. Delirium tremens is a medical emergency that requires rapid recognition and treatment
Psychotic disorder—Includes hallucinosis, paranoid states, and so called "pathological jealousy"
Amnesic syndrome—Impairment of recent memory (that is, for events that occurred a few hours previously), while both immediate recall and memories of more remote events are relatively preserved

community, but inpatient detoxification is recommended for those at risk of suicide, lacking social support, or giving a history of severe withdrawal reactions including fits and delirium tremens.

The important principles of community detoxification are:
● Daily supervision in order to allow early detection of complications such as delirium tremens, continuous vomiting, or deterioration in mental state
● The vitamin B preparation, thiamine 15 mg twice daily for three weeks, is needed to prevent Wernicke's encephalopathy. This should be given to all patients undergoing withdrawal. Severely alcohol dependent patients will need initial treatment with parental vitamins (such as Pabrinex) which, because of the risk of anaphylaxis, makes this category of patients unsuitable for a community detoxification.
● Benzodiazepines to prevent a withdrawal syndrome. The most commonly used benzodiazepine is chlordiazepoxide at a starting dose of 10 mg four times daily and reducing over seven days. Larger doses are used in severe withdrawal—for example, 40 mg four times daily reducing over 10 days. On the other hand, large doses may accumulate to dangerous levels if there is significant liver disease.

Support after withdrawal

The relapse rate among alcoholics is high but can be reduced by a programme of rehabilitation. Various options are available to assist in maintaining recovery:
● The primary healthcare team
● The community alcohol team
● Residential rehabilitation programmes
● Voluntary organisations providing support and counselling, either individually or in groups (organisations are listed in local telephone directories)
● Disulfiram has a small but useful role to play in maintaining abstinence. Patients who take disulfiram (which inhibits acetaldehyde dehydrogenase) experience the extremely unpleasant symptoms of acetaldehyde accumulation if they drink any alcohol; although usually this takes the form of vomiting, the reaction can be unpredictable and severe reactions can occur, causing collapse and requiring oxygen treatment. Controlled studies show that supervised administration, either alone or as an adjunct to psychosocial methods, is one of the few effective interventions in alcohol dependence. Abstinence rates approaching 60% at one year have been reported. There is no limit on the duration of disulfiram treatment, but liver function tests should be checked at six months as the drug itself may cause liver damage. It is contraindicated if liver disease is severe (liver enzymes over ten times normal).
● Acamprosate is a new drug licensed for use in alcohol dependence. It acts to reduce craving for alcohol probably through a direct effect on GABA receptors in the brain; unlike disulfiram it produces no adverse interaction with alcohol and so has no deterrent effect. It is a useful alternative in maintaining abstinence. It is recommended that treatment is started as soon as possible after detoxification and should be mantained even in the event of a relapse. The recommended duration of treatment is one year. Like disulfiram, it is contraindicated in severe liver disease.
● Referral to specialist mental health services for patients who show substantial psychiatric comorbidity. An important subgroup of alcoholics will require treatment for phobic anxiety or recurrent depression.

Alcohol withdrawal states

Withdrawal syndrome

Not every heavy drinker will suffer a withdrawal syndrome, but, for most who do, it is unpleasant
Onset—3-6 hours after last drink
Duration—5-7 days
Common withdrawal symptoms—Headache, nausea, vomiting, sweating and tremor. Generalised (grand mal) convulsions may occur during withdrawal

Delirium tremens

This occurs in about 5% of those suffering from alcohol withdrawal
Onset—48-72 hours or more after last drink
Features—The characteristic symptoms of delirium (agitation, confusion, visual and auditory hallucinations, and paranoia) plus the marked tremor of alcohol withdrawal
Complications—Delirium tremens is serious because of associated complications: fits, hyperthermia, dehydration, electrolyte imbalance, shock and chest infection
Prognosis—In hospital practice the mortality is high, about 10%

Chlormethiazole is no longer recommended as attenuation therapy, particularly in general practice, because of the high risk of dependence and the lethal cocktail that results if it is taken with alcohol

---

Local services

As well as mental health services, many local voluntary agencies and self help groups, such as Alcoholics Anonymous and Al-Anon, can provide much needed advice and support for patients and their families. Most voluntary agencies prefer patients to make contact directly. Details may be found in the telephone directory or *Yellow Pages*

National helplines
● DrinkLine (National Alcohol Helpline) 0345 320 202
● Sick Doctors' Trust (helpline for addicted physicians) 01252 345 163

Further reading

Chick J, Cantwell R, eds. *Seminars in alcohol and drug abuse.* London: Gaskell, 1994

Edwards G. *The treatment of drinking problems.* Oxford: Blackwell, 1987

Haig R, Hibbert G. Where and when to detoxify single homeless drinkers. *BMJ* 1990;301:848–9

Miller WR, Rollnick S. *Motivational interviewing. Preparing people to change addictive behaviour.* London: The Guildford Press, 1991

Rollnick S, Heather N, Bell A. Negotiating behaviour change in medical settings. The development of brief motivating interviewing. *J Mental Health* 1992;1:35–7

Schuckit MA. Substance use disorders. *BMJ* 1997; 314: 1605–8

Williams H, Ghodse H. The prevention of alchohol and drug misuse. In: Kendrick T, Tylee A, Freeling P, eds. *The prevention of mental illness in primary care.* Cambridge: Cambridge University Press, 1996:223–45

World Health Organization. *Alcohol action plan for Europe.* Copenhagen: WHO, 1993

UK Alcohol Forum. *Guidelines for the management of alcohol problems in primary care and general psychiatry.* High Wycombe, 1997

13 Mental health in old age

A J D Macdonald

Psychiatric care of elderly people can be more interesting than that of younger patients. Successful treatment of elderly patients requires a demanding mélange of psychological, medical, social, political, and managerial skills—an epitome of modern medicine.

Depression

> The prevalence of depression among people aged over 65 is 15% in the general community, 25% in general practice patients, and ≥30% in residential homes

Important biological symptoms of depression in old age are change in sleep patterns (especially reduced sleep and early morning wakening); decline in appetite and weight loss; regular variation of mood over day (especially worse in early morning); constipation; physical and mental slowing not accountable by other disorders; and suicidal thoughts.

The central question for doctors is whether a depressive state will respond to treatment (including electroconvulsive therapy); all other questions are either peripheral or secondary to medical practice. Social engineering is not the doctor's role. Even deciding to admit a patient to hospital is secondary to treatability: there is little point in admission if the patient, however suicidal, is unlikely to improve; better to reserve your place in the coroner's court and concentrate on more treatable patients.

The categories of depression in elderly people that respond well to treatment are
- Depression lasting more than a year—biological symptoms attenuate over time, so ask about symptoms at onset
- Depression with fixed, unreasonable beliefs of poverty, sin, guilt, persecution, filth, or dreadful internal disease or abnormality (patients particularly benefit from electroconvulsive therapy)
- Depression with hallucinations of voices haranguing, foul smells, or disgusting tastes (patients particularly benefit from electroconvulsive therapy).

Management

The mainstay of treatment is an effective antidepressant drug. Side effects are common and sometimes troublesome, but the rewards of persistence are worth while (70% of treated patients improve).

Chances of depressed patient responding to treatment

Increased if	Unaffected by
• Biological symptoms of depression prominent	• Age alone
• Record of clear change in patient's mood, however long ago	• Obvious precipitating event (such as bereavement)
• History of previous successful treatment	• Social and interpersonal difficulties (these often a consequence of depression)
• Family history of biological depression or mania	• Poverty and poor living circumstances
• No clinical evidence of dementia or from informant's history	• Intercurrent physical illness, unless terminal stages
	• Mild or moderate dementia

Criteria for hospital admission of elderly patients with depression

Those who are likely to benefit from treatment and who
- Express suicidal ideas of a definite sort, or who attempt suicide
- Have problems with compliance or delivery, leading to unduly protracted treatment
- Require electroconvulsive therapy for delusions and hallucinations
- Neglect themselves substantially, particularly their fluid intake
- Require removal from a hostile social environment
- Are in such distress as to need tranquillisation or skilled nursing care
- Have physical illness that would complicate treatment
- Harm themselves, or threaten to, for the first time (especially men)

Treatment regimen for dothiepin in elderly patients

	Bedtime dose	
	At home	In hospital or nursing home
Starting dose	25 mg	50 mg
Increment interval	7 days	5 days
Increment	25 mg	25 mg
Time to reach dose of 150 mg	42 days	20 days
Final dose	150 mg or maximum lower dose tolerated	
Check blood pressure (lying and standing)	Weekly	Every 2 days
	(Until final dose achieved for a week; thereafter only if symptoms of postural hypotension occur)	

Common side effects of dothiepin in elderly people

Symptoms	Remedy	Other problems	Remedy
Dry mouth	Fluids, lozenges	Electrocardiographic changes	Little practical importance
Constipation	Fluids, dietary fibre	Urinary hesitancy or retention	Stop: use selective serotonin reuptake inhibitor
Sweating, especially at night		Increased risk of epileptic fits	Rarely important
Drowsiness	Take drug at bedtime	Postural hypotension	Reduce dose, then cautious increase
Dizziness on standing up	Monitor blood pressure for postural hypotension	Risk of overdose	Drug very dangerous in overdose; monitor risk of suicide, prescribe frequent small script
Vivid dreams	Warning, reassurance	Worsen delirium	Do not use if risk of delirium high
Fine tremor	Reassurance		

Selective serotonin reuptake inhibitors have remarkably few side effects, are safe in overdose, and can be used as first line treatments, although they may be slow to act. The criteria for use of these drugs in elderly patients are if patients find the side effects of tricyclic antidepressants intolerable, if clinically relevant cardiac arrhythmias occur with tricyclics or are confidently predicted by an expert, in cases of poorly controlled epilepsy, in cases of depression with substantial dementia, and if the risk of delirium is high.

How long should antidepressants be continued? Although patients hate this, it seems that at least two years is the answer. Some elderly patients, especially with late onset or recurrent depression, should take antidepressants or lithium indefinitely.

Supporting the carers of depressed people

Carers need to discuss treatment and report on progress, but also need to air feelings and fears and to seek advice. Many patients leap to conclusions about the causes of their illness and plan major changes in their life (such as moving to a new home): making or allowing major life changes while a patient is depressed is folly.

Anxiety

> **The prevalence of general anxiety among people aged over 65 in the community is 4%, and the prevalence of phobias is 10%**

Anxiety in elderly people is managed exactly as in younger patients—and with equivalent success—although the circumstances may differ.

Supporting the carers of people with anxiety

Carers can be sucked into overprotection, which can wreck behavioural programmes, or adopt a self protective, indifferent attitude that hinders the patient's recovery. They need to know the consequences of their actions and attitude to the patient, and of the measures that they can take to assist the treatment programme. Again, they need the chance to express their frustrations and to feel that they are understood and appreciated—they may get little reward from the patient.

Psychotic disorders

These are conditions in which delusions (fixed, unreasonable ideas such as that neighbours are pumping noxious gas through the heating pipes) or hallucinations (such as voices plotting, commenting, or calling or strange smells or sensations) occur in the absence of substantial depression or dementia. Positive symptoms are those things (delusions and hallucinations) that "normal" people do not have. Negative symptoms are the lack of things that "normal" people do have (energy, interests, self care, reactive mood, social graces).

Acute, transient psychotic episodes are unusual in late life. More common are two categories of chronic problem with different features: persistent delusional disorder (once called "late paraphrenia") and the persistence into old age of chronic schizophrenia.

Persistent delusional disorder—In this disorder gratifying results can be seen after only a few weeks of treatment with an antipsychotic drug such as trifluoperazine, 2-5 mg thrice daily, or haloperidol, 2-10 mg daily. Use of the promising atypical antipsychotics such as olanzapine is not yet established. However, it is often the case that, although the symptoms and disturbance abate, the price is, at best, the loss of "sparkle"

How long to continue treatment with antidepressant

Category of depression	Treatment
Early onset (as in 30s), recurrent	Indefinite, with or without lithium
Late onset (as in 60s), recurrent	Indefinite, with or without lithium
Late onset, single episode	Two years

Maintenance dose of dothiepin 75 mg daily
Maintenance dose of lithium in elderly people usually in low therapeutic range (0.4-0.6 mmol/l) but may have to be higher (about 0.9 mmol/l) to work

Advice to carers of people with depression

General problems—Don't take personally; understand biological control; arrange respite from close contact; keep in touch with professional support
Anxiety—Encourage anxiety management; avoid use of stimulants and benzodiazepines
Irritability—Keep an emotional distance for duration of episode (seek support elsewhere); check when appropriate to re-engage fully
Suicidal ideas—Don't dismiss or exaggerate; call doctor if unsure of change in risk; don't take personally; reduce availability of means
Hypochondriacal ideas—Encourage only initial investigation or consultation, then discourage further consultations
Withdrawal, decline in self care—Set gentle limits and insist these are met; minimise use of substitution services (such as meals on wheels)
Excessive side effects—Know what to expect; don't collude with autonomous decisions
Desire to change life radically—Don't collude; wait until better

Special features of anxiety in elderly people

- Very often secondary to depression so inquire about depressive symptoms and, if these are present, treat depression first
- Very often caused by neglect of consequences of frightening physical illness, falls, etc, so follow up elderly people after hip fractures, falls, crime, or unexpected illnesses to make sure that agoraphobia does not become chronic
- Late onset anxiety may be a sign of early dementia so check cognitive state and accept that normal anxiety management techniques may not work as well, and that some tranquillisation (such as thioridazine) may also be necessary
- Daytime benzodiazepines almost universally cause dependence in elderly people so avoid them
- Panic disorder is sometimes difficult to distinguish from medical conditions such as paroxysmal nocturnal dyspnoea and cardiac dysrhythmias, so always examine and investigate accordingly

> **The prevalence of psychotic disorders among people aged over 65 in the community is 1%**

Psychosis in elderly people

	Onset	Positive symptoms	Treatment
Persistent delusional disorder	Old age	Common	Gratifying response
Chronic schizophrenia	Youth or middle age	Unusual	Needed initially to prevent further decline

and, at worst, the disappearance of any interest in life whatsoever. Forced intervention under the Mental Health Act should be considered only if there is substantial and prolonged distress to the patient or, which is rarely the case, definite danger to others.

Chronic schizophrenia—In contrast, chronic schizophrenia in old age is dominated by negative symptoms. Long term antipsychotic medication, sometimes by depot injection, can keep these symptoms under control and prevent the recurrence of positive ones. Old age is no bar to the use of new antipsychotic drugs such as clozapine or olanzapine.

Dementia

> The prevalence of dementia among people aged over 65 is 5% in the community and ≥80% in residential or nursing homes

Dementia is a syndrome (characteristic collection of symptoms and signs) caused by several diseases. While the syndrome is well known, hypotheses about cause have changed over time, even in the past 10 years. Received wisdom suggests that Alzheimer's disease is the most common cause, with vascular disease (mostly cerebral infarcts) second, followed by a combination of these two. New ideas include Lewy body dementia (a sort of cortical Parkinson's disease). The idea that the dementias represent an extreme of normal ageing is dead but won't lie down.

Donepezil, which apparently slows progression in Alzheimer's disease without severe side effects, is the first treatment based on the cholinergic hypothesis to become available, though protocols for its use are rudimentary. Although it was designed for mild or moderate cases of Alzheimer's disease and not other circumstances or diseases, theoretical contraindications (such as vascular or Lewy body disease) are disputed.

Assessment of dementia
The aims of medical assessment of dementia are
- To distinguish between Alzheimer's disease, vascular dementia, Lewy body disease, and the other dementing diseases (anticholinesterases may help Alzheimer's disease, anti-clotting drugs such as aspirin may prevent further damage in vascular dementia, while antipsychotics may be contraindicated in Lewy body disease)
- To identify the very rare treatable causes of dementia (as treatment may arrest the condition and hence the dementia)
- To identify any condition that can exacerbate cognitive, social, or functional impairment (such as constipation, urinary tract infection, cardiac failure, etc).

In its early stages the most reliable method of identifying any dementia, and whether Alzheimer's disease is likely, is by interviewing the patient's closest relative. Detailed psychological tests are overrated and very difficult to obtain. The search for treatable physical illnesses that can cause dementia is an esoteric and rarely rewarding activity, but other more important functions are also served by a physical examination and routine investigations.

Management of dementia
Although old age psychiatry is often seen as synonymous with managing dementia, less than half of newly referred patients have dementia. Dementia is far too big a problem to be dealt with by one specialty—most of the old health districts contained 2000-3000 cases—and the role of psychiatrists is properly confined to certain aspects of this condition. Until

Syndrome of dementia
- Decrement in memory, thinking, orientation,* comprehension, calculation, language,* judgment, social and personal relationship, self care, praxis,* and continence
- Behavioural changes such as withdrawal, decline in interests, coarsening of personality and humour, irritability, and even aggressive outbursts
- Can be preceded by depression, anxiety state, or psychosis, revealed when prodromos clears or is treated
- Progressive: "stepwise" in vascular dementia, inexorable in Alzheimer's disease
- Consciousness and awareness of surroundings remain mostly clear

* Early changes in these features more common in vascular dementia

Protocol for the routine physical investigation of cognitive impairment (delirium or dementia)
Patients of any age with rapid onset or fluctuating cognitive impairment, especially if drowsy
Full examination, investigation, and possible referral for delirium or acute confusional state

Patients aged over 75 with dementia syndromes of insidious onset
1 Collateral history (systematic inquiry)
2 Physical examination
3 No blood, urine, radiological investigations unless indicated by 1 or 2 or for possible anticholinesterase treatment of Alzheimer's disease

Patients of any age with unusual patterns of cognitive impairment in clear consciousness, or patients with onset at age under 75 years
1 Collateral history (systematic inquiry)
2 Physical examination
3 Full blood count, erythrocyte sedimentation rate, urea and electrolytes, Veneral Disease Research Laboratory test, thyroid function tests, chest x ray, urine microbiology, computed tomography of brain
4 Any further investigations suggested by 1-3

Some of the rare reversible causes of dementia syndrome*
- Hypothyroidism
- Hyperparathyroidism
- Communicating hydrocephalus
- Syphilis
- Slow growing operable cerebal tumour (not just neoplasm)
- Renal failure
- Severe depression
- Untreated schizophrenia
- Vitamin B_{12} or folic acid deficiency
- Severe anaemia in very old people
- Heavy metal or chronic anticonvulsant toxicity

* Most exacerbate non-treatable causes of dementia

Questions for relatives to detect possible early dementia
- Have you noticed any change in personality?
- Have you noticed increased forgetfulness or anxiety about forgetting things (such as using lists more, etc)?
- Have any activities been given up (hobbies and interests, shopping, dealing with finances) and why?
- Have you noticed nocturnal confusion or muddling when out of usual routine or environment, or unusual avoidance of new circumstances?
- Have you noticed surprising failure to recognise people (such as more distant relatives)?
- Have you noticed undue difficulty in speech?
- Have changes been gradual or has there been sudden worsening?

potentially effective treatments have been developed, the bulk of the work required is social in nature. However, for quixotic reasons, areas vary hugely in both the total resources available to care for those with dementia and in the balance of agencies providing them.

Voluntary organisations

- Age Concern England, Astral House, 1268 London Road, London SW16 4ER (tel 0181 679 8000)
- Alzheimer's Disease Society, Gordon House, 10 Greencoat Place, London SW1P 1PH (tel 0171 306 0606)
- Carers National Association, 20-25 Glasshouse Yard, London EC1A 4JS (tel 0171 490 8818)
- Cruse Bereavement Care, 126 Sheen Road, Richmond, Surrey TW9 1UR (tel 0181 940 4818)
- Help the Aged, St James's Walk, London EC1R 0BE (tel 0171 253 0253)

Supporting carers of people with dementia

The medical role is fairly circumscribed, but nearly every survey of carers reveals their desire for more support from their general practitioner. Most carers need a clear and sympathetic explanation of what is happening and what is likely to happen, and general practitioners, geriatricians, and psychiatrists are in the best position to provide this.

Carers need to feel that they are taken seriously and that intercurrent physical illnesses will be treated swiftly yet thoughtfully. It is a medical disgrace if this does not occur.

Delirium ("acute confusional state")

The syndrome of delirium is characterised by
- Decrement of attention, thinking, and awareness of surroundings ("clouded consciousness")
- Decrement in memory, orientation in time, and person
- Abrupt onset and markedly fluctuating course
- Visual phenomena (illusions, hallucinations) are common
- Changes in behaviour—mostly hypoactive, occasionally very disturbed and distressed.

This acute syndrome can occur during chronic dementia. It is important to recognise that abrupt worsening of a dementia may be due to a delirium, which may be caused by a treatable condition (Fig 13.1). The most common causes of delirium in elderly people are infections of the urinary tract, chest, skin, or ear; onset or exacerbation of cardiac failure; iatrogenic (nearly any drug can cause delirium, but especially psychotropic and antiparkinsonian drugs); and cerebrovascular ischaemia.

Management

Management consists of treating the underlying cause, and sometimes tranquillisation is needed to settle agitation (use thioridazine or haloperidol). Classical delirium ends either in death or in resolution (even if this is a return to pre-existing dementia). Removal of an acutely delirious patient from home to hospital may worsen the delirium, so home management is preferred.

Elder abuse

The prevalence of abuse of elderly people is unknown

British society is ageist—mental incapacity is assumed to be an inevitable consequence of aging. It follows that cruelty towards elderly people is regarded much as if they were pet animals. This intensely demeaning concept is enshrined in the

Role of old age psychiatry service in dementia

- Assessment of eligibility for treatment of Alzheimer's disease
- Assessment of need for further medical investigation (for treatable contributors or causes)
- Assessment and management of substantially disturbed behaviour (aggression, various sorts of escapology, sexual disinhibition, etc)
- Help with support and sometimes psychiatric treatment of carers
- Certain administrative functions, such as Court of Protection
- Long term day care or residential care for very disturbed patients
- Use of Mental Health Act to help assessment in difficult cases

Who does what in care of dementia

Assessment of needs—Provided by local authority
Community support (such as home help)—Provided by local authority, voluntary and private agencies
Sitting services (respite)—Provided by local authority, voluntary and private agencies
Day care (respite)—Provided by local authority, voluntary agency
Residential care (respite, permanent)—Provided by local authority, voluntary agency, private home
Medical assessment—Provided by general practitioner, geriatric services, old age psychiatry services
Management of intercurrent physical illness—Provided by general practitioner, geriatric services
Diagnosis and explanation—Provided by general practitioner, geriatric services, old age psychiatry services
Emotional support of carers—Provided by general practitioners, geriatric services, old age psychiatry services, local authority, voluntary organisations

The prevalence of delirium is 30% among elderly people admitted to hospital

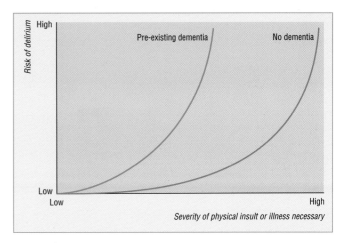

Figure 13.1 Relation of severity of insult to ease of induction of delirium

Circumstances in which abuse of people with dementia may occur

- Severe stress or frank psychiatric disorder in carer
- Intense provocation by victim's unremitting disturbed behaviour
- Ignorance of dementia (such as "He's deliberately soiling") or neglect of emotional aspects of caring
- Ignorance of strategies to deal with provocation
- Continuation of pre-existing abusive relationship
- Retribution for past unpleasantness of present victim
- Retaliation for present aggressive behaviour by victim
- Deliberate cruelty
- Exploitation for financial ends

horrific phrase "elder abuse." The real issue is abuse of anyone of whatever age who is incapable of self defence or reparation. Among elderly people, those with dementia deserve most of our attention. The risk of abuse is increased in certain circumstances, and each suggests a different response. A coordinated approach between health services, social services, and the police is now often achieved by local agencies set up specifically to this end.

Psychiatric emergencies

Elderly people may sometimes give cause for concern, and their carers may require reassurance, but genuine emergencies are relatively rare. In the following three situations, however, prompt action is necessary.

Confused person found wandering—Obtain a history from a relative or neighbour. Conduct a medical examination and perform any investigations that might be indicated. If the person is medically ill, he or she should be admitted to a medical bed, under common law if necessary. If the person is not medically ill but is still unsafe to go home (such as during winter), seek admission to emergency residential care.

Aggressive behaviour in patient with dementia—Assess "ABC" (Antecedents, Behaviour, Consequences) of circumstances in which aggression took place. If the aggressive behaviour was uncharacteristic, unprovoked, or not context specific, assess the patient for delirium. If tranquillisation is required use haloperidol or thioridazine (but not benzodiazepines). If the patient is extremely disturbed admit to an old age psychiatry ward for assessment (using the Mental Health Act if necessary).

Any serious suicide attempt or trivial suicide attempt or self harm for first time in old age—Admit the patient, especially if a man, to an old age psychiatry ward (using the Mental Health Act if necessary).

What to do about elderly people refusing treatment

As compulsory treatment can be given only in hospital, admission is the only option

Dementia and acute physical illness—Use common law to admit to care of the elderly ward

Dementia and danger to self (such as nocturnal wandering in winter)—Admit under Mental Health Act only if all reasonable alternatives (such as night sitter service) have failed; not permitted if alternatives have not been tried

Delirium but not very disturbed—Use common law to admit to care of the elderly ward

Delirium and very disturbed—Use Mental Health Act to admit

Living in squalor but no psychiatric disorder—Use section 47 of National Assistance Act only if risk to public health

Seriously physically ill but no psychiatric disorder-You may not admit compulsorily

Persecutory delusions and very distressed or dangerous to others—Use Mental Health Act to admit

Persecutory delusions but not very distressed or dangerous to others—Unwise to admit at all

Severely depressed and deluded or suicidal—Use Mental Health Act to admit

---

Further reading

British Medical Association. *Advance statements about medical treament.* London: BMJ Publishing Group, 1995

British Medical Association, the Law Society. *Assessment of mental capacity: guidance for doctors and lawyers.* London: BMA, 1995

Burns A, Harris J. Ethical issues in dementia. *Psychiar Bull* 1996; 20:107–8

14 Children and their families

Howard Roberts

Psychiatric problems in childhood are often self perpetuating and carry a substantial morbidity. In the short term they interfere with a child's emotional development, social relationships within the family and elsewhere, and with academic progress. In the long term there is an important association with adult mental illness. Child mental health services are usually provided by multidisciplinary teams: drugs are prescribed less often than in adult psychiatry, and treatments tend to be psychological with an emphasis on work with the whole family.

In infancy, a child's temperament and the quality of the relationship with the main carer (usually the mother) are important for the child's mental health. In older children, relationships within the family, success at school, and peer relationships also become important. Some children are more adaptable than others, more willing to try new experiences, or less negative when thwarted. Previous traumatic separations, physical illnesses such as asthma and cystic fibrosis, neurological problems, and developmental delay all place a child at increased risk of mental health problems. The risk is reduced if a child's family is understanding and supportive and the parents cooperate in childcare.

This chapter gives a broad overview of child mental health. Some common problems, such as difficulties with sleeping and feeding and persistent crying, are likely to be dealt with by the local health visitor or community paediatrician and have not been included here. Similarly, information on child abuse, substance misuse, and emerging sexuality are covered elsewhere.

Stages of childhood

Preschool childhood—Problems usually differ quantitatively rather than qualitatively from normal, and the severity of the symptoms is often a useful guide to their importance. Some children suffer transient reactions to upheavals in the family, such as the birth of a sibling. These tend to remit spontaneously, and all that is needed is advice and support.

Persistent problems should be identified so that help can be given. The prognosis is poorer for multiple problems, those affecting a wide aspect of a child's life and interfering with social relationships, and those that impair the ability to learn or play. Diagnostic categories used for preschool children tend to differ from those for older children.

Middle childhood—The prevalence of psychiatric problems is similar in children of school age to younger children, but diagnostic categories such as depression and obsessive-compulsive disorder become clearer and some, such as conversion disorder, appear for the first time.

Adolescence—The overall prevalence of psychiatric problems remains similar, but the clinical syndromes increasingly resemble those of adult life. Depression, anxiety, and conduct disorder, or a mixture of these, are most common, while developmental disorders, enuresis, and encopresis are much less frequent. Schizophrenia, affective psychosis, suicide, and parasuicide may be diagnosed for the first time, and there is a large increase in the prevalence of substance misuse and anorexia nervosa.

Prevalence of mental health problems in childhood

Most psychiatric disorders of childhood are more common in boys than girls.
- 15% of children in inner city areas
- 5-8% of children in rural areas
- 20% of children attending a general practitioner have psychological problems—usually presenting as physical complaints
- 30% of children attending paediatric clinics have psychiatric problems—either alone or coexisting with their physical illness
- 2.5% of school age children and 4.5% of adolescents suffer depression
- 7% of three year olds in London were found to have moderate to severe behaviour problems. Two-thirds of those with generalized problems at age three had problems at home and at school at four and eight years
- 4% of 10-11 year olds in the Isle of Wight study showed conduct disorder, with a higher prevalence in urban areas.

Many of these childhood disorders are undiagnosed and untreated

---

Maternal care-giving

Quality of maternal care depends on:
- The mother's own childhood experiences
- Support she receives from her partner
- Existence of other social supports
- Compatibility between her temperament and that of her child
- Presence of mental health problems (such as depression)

Although the main caregiver is usually the mother, the father has been found to be the primary attachment figure for about one-third of 18 month old children

---

Psychiatric problems in pre-school children

Emotional problems—Such as misery, apathy, fears and worries
Behavioural problems—Such as defiance, disobedience, aggression, destructiveness, restlessness, poor concentration
Developmental disorders—Such as speech delay
Other problems—Such as soiling, sleeping problems, head banging and failure to thrive

---

Developmental problems

Learning disability is termed mental retardation in the World Health Organization's classification and is defined as "arrested or incomplete development of the mind." Diagnosis is based on the use of age standardised intelligence tests, together with an assessment of the global level of a patient's abilities. Mentally retarded people have a high prevalence of other mental disorders and of epilepsy.

Specific developmental problems include delays in achieving motor milestones or acquiring skills. Sometimes clumsiness is associated with difficulties in planning and organising. Parents are often the first to notice this, and it can be persistent resulting in a sense of failure. Language problems should be referred for a full assessment—to exclude environmental deprivation, deafness, or autism—and language therapy.

Autism is a pervasive developmental disorder with abnormalities in verbal and non-verbal communication, and social interaction. It is uncommon, and the child should be referred for specialist assessment.

Emotional disorders

Anxiety

Anxiety is part of normal development but is pathological if it is severe or persistent or occurs at an inappropriate age. Infants begin to show a fear of strangers at about 7 months; at about 9 months, they protest if separated from their carers; and 1-2 year olds become anxious if left, but less so if they initiate the separation. Specific fears peak at about age 5 and then decline: 2 year olds often fear strange objects and people; at 3 years, they fear animals; and at 4-5, they fear the dark.

Separation anxiety—Clinical features include distress on separation from the mother or main carer, worries about family members, clinging, refusal to go to school. General practitioners can minimise this problem by encouraging pleasurable separations from the mother and multiple attachments to other adults. Severe cases require behaviour therapy plus family therapy and psychodynamic individual therapy.

Social anxiety—A child is shy and withdrawn, anxious with strangers, and seeks the presence of familiar people. General practitioners can help by discouraging the avoidance of social situations and helping with social skills. Severe cases require behaviour therapy, with or without family therapy.

Phobic anxieties are irrational fears that may continue into adult life. Behavioural treatments such as modelling (in which the therapist "models" approaching the feared object), cognitive therapy (to reduce thoughts that tend to exacerbate the phobias), and desensitisation are used.

Overanxious disorder—Anxiety may not be focused on any particular object or situation but presents as fears, nightmares, loss of self confidence, seeking approval, apprehensiveness, multiple somatic complaints, and refusal to go to school. The parents may be chronically anxious. General practitioners can help by discouraging irrational negative thoughts and helping the child and parents to reinterpret situations in more positive ways. In severe cases individual, family, or behaviour therapy may be needed.

Depression

Depression is uncommon in preschool children, but the prevalence increases to adult levels during adolescence, when suicide and parasuicide occur for the first time. Depression is underdiagnosed, as parents tend to be unaware of their child's symptoms. In clinic samples childhood depression is a chronic condition with high rates of relapse, but this may not apply to

---

Developmental disorders

Mental retardation—Severity is based on the IQ derived from standardised intelligence tests: mild (IQ 50-69), moderate (IQ 35-49), severe (IQ 20-34), profound (IQ < 20). The term learning disability is often preferred

Pervasive developmental disorders—Development is abnormal throughout infancy, and the full disorder is apparent before the age of 5. Includes childhood autism and Asperger's syndrome

Specific developmental disorders of speech and language—These include specific delays in articulation and speech sound production, expressive language use, and receptive understanding of language

Specific developmental disorders of scholastic skills—The inability to acquire specific skills (reading, spelling or arithmetic) despite the absence of gross brain disease and ample opportunity for learning. Often follows earlier developmental delays. Includes dyslexia or backward reading

Specific developmental disorder of motor function—Seriously impaired development of motor control, often with soft neurological signs, but no specific neurological disorder. Includes clumsy child syndrome

---

Emotional disorders of childhood

Most emotional disorders specific to childhood have a prominent anxiety component

Separation anxiety disorder
- Characterised by a preoccupying fear that the child will be separated from his or her carer. May involve fears of the carer's or the child's loss, injury or death
- Associated with disturbed sleep and nightmares, refusal to attend school, and somatic complaints
- May represent a persistence of normal separation anxiety or may be precipitated by acute stress or separation at a later age
- Improves with age but may worsen in adolescence, and many adults with agoraphobia have a history of separation anxiety disorder

Social anxiety disorder
- A persistent fear and avoidance of strangers, and social interactions, arising before the age of 6 years
- Includes avoidant disorder of childhood.
- Spontaneous improvement is unlikely, and it may lead to social phobia

Phobic anxiety disorder
- Fear focused on a particular object (open or closed spaces, animals, heights, the dark, thunder, school, etc)
- Arises during an appropriate developmental phase, but excessive for that phase

Sibling rivalry disorder
- Persistent negative feelings which arise soon after the birth of a younger sibling, and ranging from a lack of friendly interactions to hostility with physical or psychological trauma

Other childhood emotional disorders
- Includes overanxious disorder and identity disorder

Depression in childhood

Symptoms of depression in children are similar to those experienced by adults

Depression is under-diagnosed because
- Parents are unaware of child s symptoms
- Child is unable to articulate his or her symptoms
- Doctor (or others) do not believe children become depressed
- Child not interviewed alone, or not given opportunity to express symptoms

community samples. Follow up studies indicate some continuity between childhood depression and depression in adult life.

Undesirable life events such as bereavement and divorce increase the risk of depression, although most children exposed to such events do not become depressed. Children subject to abuse or bullying at school are more likely to become depressed. They may find it difficult to talk about these problems, and some try to conceal them. A poor relationship with the mother increases the risk of depression, as does parental depressive illness. Depressed children may be anxious or aggressive and often have poor peer relationships and problems at school. In adolescence depression becomes much more common in girls, a pattern that continues into adult life.

Treatment—It is important to interview the child alone. It may be enough to offer supportive family therapy and remove environmental stresses. More severe cases need psychotherapy to increase the child's self confidence and reduce negative cognitions. Treating children with antidepressant drugs remains controversial.

Emotional problems presenting with somatic symptoms

Children often present with physical symptoms with no organic cause, which may indicate that they are unable to express emotional distress in words. Other family members may also have unexplained physical symptoms. Abdominal and head pain are the most common symptoms, but several other, less common somatic presentations also occur.

Treatment—The tasks are to identify stresses, help the child and the family redefine the symptoms in psychological terms, and help them find a way of resolving the child's predicament. A child with chronic fatigue syndrome will require both psychological and physical rehabilitation: maladaptive ideas about the illness may respond to cognitive therapy, and antidepressants sometimes help. Cognitive therapy may help in treating body dysmorphic disorder. With conversion disorder, chronic fatigue syndrome, and somatisation disorder, the family may be hostile to psychological explanations for the symptoms. In such cases it is important to gain the parents' cooperation before starting treatment and to avoid disputes about the need for psychiatric help.

Obsessive-compulsive disorder

Obsessional symptoms, such as jumping over cracks between paving stones, are common in preschool children and are part of normal development. Obsessive-compulsive disorder is uncommon at all ages, but prevalence increases at school age and again in adolescence.

The symptoms resemble those in adults, and may be so severe that children may stop attending school. Often they cannot keep their obsessions to themselves and manipulate their family into fitting in with their anxieties. Despite this, children are often referred only after symptoms have been present for years. In about two thirds of adults with obsessive-compulsive disorder the symptoms started in adolescence.

Treatment with fluoxetine or clomipramine, under specialist guidance, may be combined with family behaviour therapy to reduce the family's collusion in maintaining symptoms.

Enuresis

Non-organic enuresis is primary if a child has never been dry and secondary if he or she starts to wet again after achieving continence. Daytime continence is usually attained first, and most children become dry at night at 2-4 years old: it is therefore unusual to diagnose or treat enuresis until after the age of 5. Children who have been dry may become incontinent after a period of stress or illness.

Risk factors for depression in children

- Undesirable life events, such as bereavement and parents' divorce
- Exposure to physical, sexual, or emotional abuse or bullying at school
- Poor relationship with mother or main carer
- Parental depressive illness
- Anxiety or aggression, and often poor peer relationships and problems at school
- Female (adolescence)

Emotional problems presenting with somatic symptoms

Abdominal pain
- Occurs in about 10% of children, the rate increasing from 3-9 years and then declining
- Pain may be associated with social stress: some children are depressed, anxious and fearful, while others have behavioural problems and temper tantrums
- A child may be over-dependent, and pain may show a temporal pattern which coincides with separations such as school attendance.
- The pain may remit within a few months or become chronic

Headaches
- Common at all ages
- A child may admit to being under stress, or come from an enmeshed family where the expression of emotion is difficult
- In affected adolescents, there is sometimes a conflict between desire to achieve independence and guilt at breaking away from the family

Conversion disorder
- A loss or alteration of physical functioning suggestive of a physical disorder—which may be dramatic such as hemiplegia
- Often occurs when a child has an unresolvable conflict, such as bereavement, and the symptoms may resemble those of the person who has died
- Occurs in association with sexual abuse, but a precipitant cannot always be identified
- Families often antagonistic to psychological explanations

Chronic fatigue syndrome
- Symptoms similar to those in adults
- In many cases the symptoms remit but these children can become chronically disabled

Body dysmorphic disorder
- The symptom of "imagined ugliness" is uncommon, but affected children may request surgery to correct their perceived cosmetic defects
- Some children have bizarre ideas about their appearance, and there may be an underlying depression

Somatisation disorder
- Children sometimes present with multiple somatic complaints resembling those in adults

Treatment—A simple method is to allow unrestricted fluids during the day, while teaching the child to practise deferring micturition, then restricting fluids before bedtime and waking the child at night to pass urine. "Star charts" to record successes produce marked improvement in 20% of cases. Studies using a night alarm report a success rate of about 80%. Desmopressin, a synthetic analogue of vasopressin with antidiuretic but little vasopressor effects, may be useful. It can be administered as a nasal spray and has few side effects. Tricyclic antidepressants offer brief symptom relief, but they may cause cardiac side effects. Relapse is common when any drug treatment is stopped.

Conduct disorder

This consists of persistent behavioural problems that violate social norms appropriate to the child's age, including aggression, stealing, lying, and running away. It is more common in boys than girls and often occurs in preschool children, where it is associated with developmental delay, language delay, overactivity, and anxiety. Its prevalence rises in adolescence and declines in early adulthood. However, there is continuity between aggression and dissocial behaviour in childhood, adolescence, and adult life, and aggressive children are at increased risk of delinquency and drug misuse.

Features—The family may be unable to set rules, monitor behaviour, or reward socially acceptable behaviour, and parents may be lax or excessively punitive. Onset may be linked to an acute stress such as bereavement. A child may be impulsive, inconsistent, and violent; have few social skills; and show high levels of anxiety and conflict. He or she may show cognitive problems, be likely to misinterpret the intentions of others as hostile, and have difficulty solving social problems. As a consequence, he or she is more likely to use violence. There is a high rate of depression and an important link with reading retardation.

Treatment—It is important to work with the family to alleviate stresses on the child and to create a secure, consistent environment where socially acceptable behaviour is rewarded. The tendency to misinterpret others' behaviour may respond to cognitive therapy, social skills training, or psychodynamic therapy. Reading retardation and other developmental delays need specific treatment.

Hyperkinetic disorders

These disorders are much more common in boys than in girls. They are usually diagnosed in the early school years, but about half such children show overactivity before they are 4 years old. Parents usually complain of management difficulties, and the relationship between mother (or main carer) and child can become very negative.

At school, teachers find it difficult to keep the child on task, the child cannot concentrate and falls behind with work, and a cycle of negative, attention seeking behaviour may be established. As the child grows older, he may become increasingly aware of these problems. Prognosis is poor, and follow up studies of hyperkinetic preschool children show that half have behavioural problems (mainly dissocial personality disorder, drug misuse, or criminality) in adult life.

Treatment—Methylphenidate improves the child's symptoms and reduces the negativity of the interaction between mother and child. However, medication may not improve the long term prognosis. Behavioural interventions with the mother may improve the child's symptoms and the mother-child interaction, but it is uncertain whether this produces long term benefits.

Bladder and bowel control

Bladder and bowel problems can result in a very tense, punitive relationship between child and parent which tends to increase the child's anxiety and thus perpetuate the problem.

Nonorganic enuresis
- Investigation of the urinary tract should be considered if daytime wetting continues after the age of 3 years

Nonorganic encopresis
- Passage of normal-looking faeces at inappropriate times or places, at an age when normal bowel control would be expected
- Usually accompanied by emotional or behavioural disturbances and may involve deliberately depositing or smearing the faeces over the child's body or surroundings
- Encopresis and enuresis may occur together, and organic causes should be excluded.

Conduct disorders

Types
- Dissocial or aggressive behaviour may occur entirely within the family, or may pervade all aspects of the child's world
- It may be unsocialised (in which the child is solitary, and lacks close relationships) or socialised (where the child has developed close, lasting and loyal friendships with other—often normal—children)
- Oppositional defiant disorder is characterised by marked defiant and disobedient behaviour in the absence of severe dissocial or aggressive behaviour or law breaking

Associated mental health problems
- Developmental delays (including language and reading); overactivity, anxiety, depression; brain damage
- Cognitive problems—Interprets behaviour of other people as hostile; cannot think of non-violent ways of solving social problems; poor social skills and interactions

Family factors
- Failure to set appropriate limits and monitor behaviour; failure to reward socially acceptable behaviour
- Inconsistent discipline
- Violent role models
- Family conflict

Hyperkinetic disorders

Clinical features
- Grossly impaired attention and overactivity are present in all areas of the child's life
- There may be difficulty in concentrating, distractibility, impulsiveness, restlessness, and, in some situations, recklessness and social disinhibition
- Child may be "accident-prone" or "troublesome" rather than actively defiant

Associated problems
- Developmental delays, reading difficulties, and other scholastic problems
- Child may seem domineering or aggressive and be unpopular with his or her peers
- There may also be a coexisting conduct disorder

Hyperkinetic disorders include disorders previously termed attention deficit hyperactivity disorder (ADHD).

Eating disorders

Anorexia nervosa is uncommon in prepubertal children and is most common in adolescent girls (peak age of onset 14-18 years); it is rarer and more serious in boys. Symptoms include reduced eating, weight loss, amenorrhoea, and disturbance in body image. Mortality is lower than in adults, but about a third of affected children have psychiatric symptoms such as depression, obsessive-compulsive disorder, or social phobia at follow up.

Bulimia nervosa shows a similar sex distribution, although the age of onset may be later. It may become established as a sequel to anorexia.

Treatment is by combined family and individual therapy.

Psychoses

Schizophrenia and affective psychoses are rare before puberty and become commoner in adolescence. Although the symptoms may resemble those in adults, it may be difficult to distinguish between the two conditions in this age group. The poor prognosis of early onset disorders may be improved by prompt treatment, and the main factors affecting outcome seem to be premorbid functioning and degree of recovery from a first episode.

Treatment is the same as in adults, but family therapy has an important place. Children may have a higher rate of side effects with antipsychotic drugs than adults. The newer "a typical" antipsychotic drugs such as clozapine and risperidone have not been fully evaluated in children.

I am grateful to Dr Peter Loader for his helpful comments.

Anorexia nervosa

Self-induced weight loss—Dieting, vomiting, purging, diuretic misuse, excessive exercise

Low body weight—At least 15% lower than expected; body mass index (weight (kg)/height (m)^2) of ≤ 17.5

Body image distortion—An overvalued idea of being "fat"

Endocrine abnormalities—Delayed puberty in prepubertal children, amenorrhoea in girls, lack of sexual interest in boys. Growth hormone, cortisol, insulin and thyroid hormone levels may all be affected

---

Bulimia nervosa

This shares many psychopathological features with anorexia nervosa, and the pattern of overeating and vomiting may occur as sequel to anorexia nervosa.

Preoccupation with eating—Craving for food, "binge eating"

Abnormal weight maintenance—Periods of starvation; repeated vomiting; misuse of purgatives, diuretics, and other weight or appetite modulating drugs

Morbid ideas—Dread of being "fat"

Electrolyte abnormalities—Repeated vomiting may induce physical disorder (such as seizures, cardiac dysrhythmias)

Comorbidity—Depressive symptoms, self harm, drug or alcohol misuse, personality disorder

---

Further reading

Black D, Cottrell D. *Seminars in child and adolescent psychiatry*. London: Gaskell, 1993.

Goodman R. Child mental health: who is responsible? *BMJ* 1997;314:813-817.

Department of Health. *A handbook on child and adolescent mental health*. Leeds: NHS Executive, 1995.

Kurtz Z, Thornes R, Wolkind S. *National survey of mental health services for children and young people. Report to the Department of Health*. London: DoH, 1994.

Lawrenson F. Runaway children: whose problem? *BMJ* 1997;314:1064.

Levy F. Attention deficit hyperactivity disorder. *BMJ* 1997;315:894-5.

15   Mental health in a multiethnic society

Simon Dein

People from ethnic minorities comprise just over three million people or 5.5% of the British population. Their geographical distribution is highly uneven, with most living in greater London, the West Midlands, and other metropolitan counties.

Doctors in Britain increasingly encounter patients whose values and beliefs differ substantially from their own. Without a knowledge of other cultural beliefs and practices, doctors can easily fall prey to errors of diagnosis, resulting in inappropriate management and poor compliance. For example, a delusion is a false belief not amenable to reason and out of context with a person's cultural and religious beliefs: diagnosing someone as deluded must take into account cultural and religious factors.

Culture refers to the categories, plans, and rules that people use to interpret their world and act purposefully within it. These rules are learned in childhood while growing up in society. Cultural factors relate to mental illness in several ways. In the first instance, culture determines what is seen as normal and abnormal within a given society.

Normal and abnormal behaviour

Definitions of what constitutes normal and abnormal behaviour vary widely from culture to culture and, within any given group, are dependent on demographic factors such as age and sex, social class, and occupation. Behaviours that may be perceived as abnormal at one time may be regarded as normal at other times, such as during carnivals. At these times it is culturally acceptable for men to dress as women or animals.

However, it seems that there is no culture in which men and women remain oblivious to erratic, disturbed, threatening, or bizarre behaviour in their midst. This is the more so when such behaviours occur without reason. In some cultures these behaviours may be seen as bad, meriting punishment, while in others they may be seen as signs of illness requiring treatment.

Idioms of distress

British doctors may encounter behaviours that in other societies are acceptable, at least sometimes, but that could be interpreted as signs of mental illness: witchcraft and possession states are good examples of this. In many parts of the world these are culturally sanctioned ways of accounting for misfortune or expressing distress and are socially acceptable as such.

Obeah

A prevalent belief among immigrants from rural (and sometimes urban) communities of Africa and Asia is that it is possible to influence the health or wellbeing of another person by action at a distance. Culturally sanctioned ways of dealing with this often involve resorting to traditional healers or the use of counter-magic. Among Afro-Caribbean people in Britain a belief in obeah is common, and various countermeasures are employed.

A doctor presented with someone claiming to have been bewitched may misdiagnose a paranoid disorder and treat the patient with antipsychotic drugs. Involving a traditional healer would be more appropriate, and, in the absence of a suitable healer, a Christian priest might be acceptable since many believers in witchcraft also adhere to Christianity.

Ethnic composition of Great Britain in 1991*

| Ethnic group† | Population (1000s) | Percentage of population | |
		Of total (54 889 000)	Of ethnic minority
White	51 874	94.5	
All ethnic minorities	3 015	5.5	100
Black:	891	1.6	29.5
Caribbean	500	0.9	16.6
African	212	0.4	7.0
Other	178	0.3	5.9
South Asian:	1 480	2.6	49.1
Indian	840	1.5	27.9
Pakistani	477	0.8	15.8
Bangladeshi	163	0.3	5.4
Chinese and others:	645	1.1	21.4
Chinese	157	0.3	5.2
Other Asian	198	0.4	6.6
Other non-Asian	290	0.5	9.6

*Data from Commission for Racial Equality
†Categories according to Office for Population Censuses and Surveys

---

"Culture is that complex whole which includes knowledge, beliefs, art, morals, law, customs, etc"
Definition of culture, Tyler 1874

Culture relates to mental illness in several ways, especially its mode of presentation and response to treatment

---

"Obeah" is a form of witchcraft containing elements of Christianity, animism, folk medicine, and personal malevolence

---

Culturally appropriate reactions may be misdiagnosed as mental illness

Miss E, a 20 year old woman who had emigrated to Britain from Trinidad, was compulsorily admitted to hospital after refusing food and drink for several days.

She believed that an obeah curse had been placed on her. A diagnosis was made of severe psychotic depression and treatment commenced under the emergency provisions of the Mental Health Act.

Response to treatment was poor, and a traditional healer was consulted, who lifted the curse. She began to eat and drink and showed no other signs of mental illness; she was discharged from hospital two days later.

Possession

This means the takeover of a person's mind and body by an external force such as a spirit or ancestor. The force controls the patient's thoughts and actions and deprives him or her of responsibility for these actions. In many parts of the world people freely admit to being possessed and to having spirits speak and act through them. Anthropologists point out that this mode of expression is deployed by disadvantaged members of a group to gain otherwise unattainable ends. The possessed person seems to be in a trance-like state and may perform actions that are totally out of character (Fig 15.1).

This state may be misdiagnosed as schizophrenia and treated as such. However, a more satisfactory outcome is likely if an exorcism is performed by the religious authorities, while the doctor should pay attention to the interpersonal problems in the patient's family that are likely to have been the precipitants.

Explanations of mental illness

Each culture provides its members with ways of explaining mental illness, attempting to answer questions about why, and under what circumstances, someone becomes mentally ill. In the West emphasis is placed on psychological factors, life events, and the effects of stress, but in many parts of the Third World explanations of mental illness take into account wider social and religious factors. These include spirit possession, witchcraft, the breaking of religious taboos, divine retribution, and the capture of the soul by a spirit. Thus, these factors may need to considered if treatment is to be accepted. For example, taking tablets may not make sense to a patient who perceives his or her problems to lie in some religious misdemeanour.

Presentation of mental illness

Evidence from studies by transcultural psychiatrists and psychologists indicates that the major mental disorders, schizophrenia and depressive illness, occur worldwide.

Schizophrenia—Although the form of the disorder remains constant, culture determines the content of the illness and the way that it is expressed. Delusions and hallucinations draw on the symbols and images of the patient's cultural milieu. For example, in the West delusions often relate to technology (such as electricity being put into the brain, or being controlled by computer), while in Africa and India it is more common for delusions to have a religious basis (involving being taken over or harmed by gods or spirits).

Depression—Among people from the Far East and from lower socioeconomic groups in Western cultures, depressive illness may present primarily as physical symptoms (somatisation). Patients from such backgrounds might complain of lethargy and joint pains rather than low mood. Failure to recognise the underlying depression may result in patients being subjected to unnecessary physical investigations, prolonging the symptoms and reinforcing beliefs in their physical nature. Such symptoms are likely to respond to conventional antidepressant treatments.

Culture bound syndromes

These are culturally determined abnormal behaviour patterns that are specific to a particular culture or geographical region. The behaviours express core cultural themes and have a wide range of symbolic meanings—social, moral, and psychological. It is debatable how these disorders relate to conventional Western categories of mental illness. However, disorders recognised in the West such as anorexia nervosa, agoraphobia, and parasuicide may also be regarded as culture bound syndromes expressing notions of the role of women in Western society.

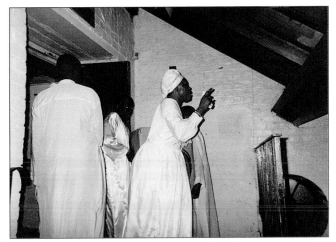

Figure 15.1   West Indian Pentecostalist possessed by the Holy Spirit. While in this state the prophetess can speak in tongues. This may be mistaken for psychotic behaviour

---

Patient and doctor may hold conflicting explanatory models of illness

Mr C, a 30 year old Vietnamese patient, had suffered from schizophrenia for 10 years. He was extremely reluctant to accept depot antipsychotic drugs and suffered frequent relapses.

Discussions with him and his family, aided by an interpreter, revealed that they believed he was possessed by evil spirits. Since this was essentially a religious problem, they believed that drugs would be of no help.

This revelation did not immediately improve his compliance with treatment, but it provided a better understanding of his reluctance and increased his (and his family's) trust in his doctor

---

> The prognosis of schizophrenia is better in Third World societies than in Western ones, and this may relate to support from families who share the patient's beliefs

---

Depression may present with somatic symptoms

Mr K, a 52 year old married man from Delhi, had lived in Britain for over 20 years.

He presented to his general practitioner with a two month history of lethargy, weakness, and aching joints. He was subjected to several physical investigations, but no abnormality was detected.

When he was interviewed by a Hindi-speaking doctor he admitted to low mood, poor appetite, and anhedonia. A diagnosis of depressive disorder was made and he responded well to conventional antidepressant drugs

---

Culture bound syndromes

These are syndromes of behaviours or beliefs that are specific to certain cultures and reflect core cultural themes

Amok—A spree of sudden violent attacks on people, animals, or property affecting men in Malaysia

Koro—A belief that the penis is shrinking into the abdomen

Evil Eye—A belief among Latin Americans that illness is caused by the stare of a jealous person

Susto—A belief in the loss of the soul in Latin America

Latah—Syndrome of increased suggestibility and imitative behaviour found in South East Asia

Migration and mental disorder

Most studies of psychiatric disorder among immigrants to Britain are based on hospital admission records. West Indian immigrants have higher admission rates for schizophrenia than people born in Britain, although there has been concern that this may be accounted for in part by overdiagnosis of schizophrenia in this group. Similarly, the rate of schizophrenia in immigrants from West Africa aged 25-35 has been estimated at nearly 30 times that of the native British population. While about 8% of white patients in psychiatric hospitals are detained under the Mental Health Act, the figure for black patients is about 25%. Men from Northern Ireland are more likely to be admitted with a diagnosis of alcoholism than native British men.

Of course, these statistics have major pitfalls and may not reflect the true prevalence of the disorders in these populations. Factors such as stigmatisation and racism are likely to account for some of the differences in admission rates.

Two theories have been proposed to account for the purported high prevalence of mental disorder among immigrants. The first is that people who are mentally ill are the ones most likely to emigrate; the second is that the stress of migration results in mental breakdown. There seems to be no single explanation for the differing rates of mental illness that is applicable to all minority or ethnic groups. Without doubt, factors such as dislocation from the native community, rejection by the host community, and difficulties in adapting to the cultural norms of the host society are perceived as intensely stressful and may contribute to mental breakdown in some vulnerable individuals.

Family structure

Norms of family structure may differ from those in the West. Asian immigrants to Britain may have extended families, in which couples and their children may live under one roof with grandparents, aunts, uncles, and nieces. Concepts of respect and disrespect, loyalty, independence, position of elders, and obligations to the family and to the wider community all vary between different ethnic groups.

Conflicts arising between family members reflect this complexity. For example, the marriages of most Indian and Pakistani adults now resident in Britain were arranged for them by their parents. Often, one partner arrived from the home country just before the marriage ceremony while the other had been brought up in Britain. Such partners are likely to hold very different value systems, which, together with the obligation to honour their families' expectations, may place their marriage under considerable strain and lead to marital breakdown.

Psychosexual disorders

The prevalence of psychosexual disorders among ethnic minorities in Britain is unknown, but it seems likely that most of these disorders are treated by indigenous healers. A common complaint by men from the Indian subcontinent is that sperm is leaking from the body into the urine. This complaint—called "jiryan" in Pakistan and "dhat" in India—may be prompted by anxiety over sexual potency or guilt about masturbation, and it may be compounded by cloudiness of the urine secondary to infection. It may also be used to explain various other problems due to organic disease or feelings of depression. It is important to recognise that this is not a delusion but a widely held belief.

Cultural aspects of treatment

The first step in treating patients from ethnic minority groups is, as with all patients, to decide if a problem exists and, if it does, to clarify its nature and degree. The general principles of

Hospital admission for schizophrenia by country of birth★

	Men	Women
England	9	9
Ireland	18	22
Caribbean	39	35
India	11	18
Pakistan	19	12

★ Rates of hospital admission per 100 000 of each population over a period of 15 years (includes paranoid psychoses). Data from Cochrane R, Bal SS. Migration and schizophrenia: an examination of five hypotheses. *Social Psychiatry* 1987; 22: 181–91

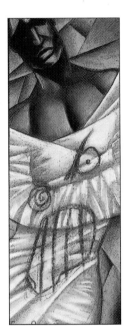

Marital and family therapy for ethnic minorities must take into account cultural aspects of family structure or they risk creating their own problems. A family therapist's encouragement to a teenage daughter to strive for self fulfilment may be in direct conflict with the father's views of the authority of the male head of the family and his notion of good conduct

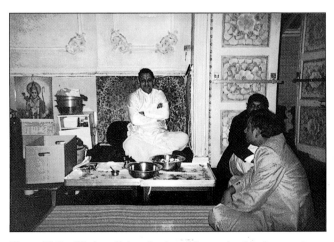

Figure 15.2 Hindu religious healer: sick people visit the temple to commune with the gods

this process apply to all patients, but to these should be added a knowledge of the culture from which a patient derives. It is important to remember that, for many people from ethnic minorities, their everyday experience of racism is a major factor shaping their presentation and use of health services.

It is vital to find out how a patient seems to members of his or her own culture, and a doctor is likely to benefit from enlisting the help of the patient's family and close friends. Other useful, and often important, informants include religious officials and traditional healers, together with an interpreter when there are linguistic problems. It is, of course, important to be aware that an interpreter (especially if a member of the patient's family) may have a vested interest in presenting the patient as mad if the patient has broken a taboo, has been sexually promiscuous, or is resisting family pressures.

It may be decided that a mental health problem does not exist and that the "patient" is exhibiting culturally appropriate behaviour. In this case, a traditional healer may be more relevant than a general practitioner or psychiatrist. Traditional healers are better at treating certain problems than Western practitioners. For example, hakims (Moslem) and vaids (Hindu) (Fig 15.2) may be better at dealing with psychosexual problems in their community than conventional psychosexual therapists.

When a mental disorder is recognised and it is appropriate to apply Western treatments such as drugs or electroconvulsive therapy, it is still important to elicit the patient's own explanatory model of the illness and attempt to explain the treatment in these terms. This will enhance the patient's trust in the doctor and improve compliance.

Other factors affecting treatment
More work is needed on the different response to psychotropic drugs among different ethnic groups. It seems that south Asian patients show higher plasma concentrations of antidepressants than do white patients given a similar dose. These patients may be more sensitive to side effects and respond to lower doses.

Transcultural psychiatrists have found that management of mental illness in the Third World must take into account not only the patient but the wider kinship group of which the patient is a member. Treatment aims to resolve tensions among family members, which may have been causally related to the patient's illness. Psychiatric management of disorders among ethnic minorities in Britain must also take account of these factors.

Intercultural therapy
Several centres have been established in Britain to provide psychotherapy to ethnic minority groups. Among the best known is the Nafsiyat Inter-Cultural Therapy Centre in north London. It is funded jointly by the local authority and the health service and offers formal psychotherapy to members of ethnic minority groups, taking account of racial and cultural components in mental disorder. It is involved in organising training courses and seminars in intercultural therapy and in conducting research into the efficacy of treatment.

The artwork is by Tracy Cox and reproduced with permission of the Stock Illustration Source.

Making mental health services more accessible for ethnic minorities
Patients
- To be treated with respect
- To be interviewed by staff with relevant language skills, or accompanied by an interpreter
- To be encouraged to explain their views, and to have the views of the doctor explained to them

Doctors and other staff
- To understand issues of racism and stigma in relation to the mental health of ethnic minority groups
- To be aware of, and be instructed in, the cultural norms and religious beliefs of the main ethnic groups consulting them
- To elicit and attempt to understand the explanatory models of illness used by their patients, and to consider the value of traditional healing methods

Ethnic minority groups
- To be provided with information about Western concepts of mental illness and its treatments
- To be consulted and involved in developing services
- To be encouraged to join patient support and advocacy groups

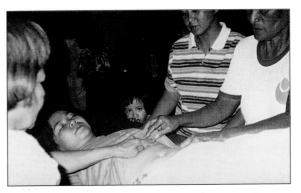

Figure 15.3 A Filipino psychic surgeon about to perform a psychic operation. This involves the supposed removal of tumours and tissues without the use of anaesthetic and leaving no scar

Agencies providing mental health services for ethnic minorities
- African Caribbean Mental Health Association (tel 0171 737 3603) provides advice, counselling and psychotherapy for individuals, families, and groups
- Fanon Centre, Brixton, London (tel 0171 737 2888) is a drop-in and advice centre for mentally ill people of Afro-Caribbean origin. It has support groups for women, homeless people, and families
- Ipamo ("A place of healing," tel 0171 737 4585) is a developing alternatives to hospital admission for black people with mental health problems
- Nafsiyat Inter-Cultural Therapy Centre, 278 Seven Sisters Road, London N4 (tel 0171 263 4130)
- Vietnamese Mental Health Project (tel 0171 326 5565) provides support for Vietnamese refugees and their families

Further reading
Bhui K, Christie Y, Bhugra D. Essential elements in culturally sensitive psychiatric services. *Int J Soc Psychiatry* 1995;41:242–56
Cole E, Leavey G, King M, Johnson-Sabine E, Hoar A. Pathways to care for patients with a first episode of psychosis. A comparison of ethnic groups. *Br J Psychiatry* 1995; 167:770–6
King M, Coker E, Leavey G, Hoare A, Johnson-Sabine E. Incidence of psychotic illness in London: comparison of ethnic groups. *BMJ* 1994;309:1115–9
NHS Executive Mental Health Task Force. *Black mental health—a dialogue for change.* London: Department of Health, 1994
Singh SP. Ethnicity in psychiatric epidemiology: need for precision. *Br J Psychiatry* 1997; **171**:305–8
Yee L. *Improving support for black carers. A source book of information, ideas and initiatives.* London: Kings Fund, 1995

16 Mental health on the margins

Philip Timms, John Balázs

Mental illness and homelessness

People with mental illness have always been marginalised and economically disadvantaged, and deprived inner city areas have excessive rates of severe mental illness. Homelessness is the most marginalised end of the spectrum of poverty, and here are found disproportionate numbers of mentally ill people.

Homeless people do not constitute a homogenous population: disparate groups have widely differing needs. The mental health needs of people living in "traditional" homeless lifestyles have elicited particular concern. We focus on the situation in Britain, but similar problems exist in most Western industrialised nations.

Size of the problem

Reliable estimates of the numbers of homeless people are notoriously dificult to come by. The 1991 census concluded that about 3000 people were sleeping out and 20,000 were living in hostels for the homeless, but these figures are now recognised to have been underestimates. In addition, 169,966 households were registered as statutorily homeless in 1992.

Although the absolute numbers are small, homeless people place disproportionately large demands on services. Compared with the general population, at least twice as many homeless people have some kind of important mental health problem.

Nature of the problem

There are no mental illnesses or emotional problems unique to homeless people. They suffer from the same disorders as the general population, but there are three main differences.

Prevalence of all mental disorders is higher. Psychosis is overrepresented by a factor of 20 or 30 in hostel populations.

Social support and resources that are necessary for health, and taken for granted by most people, simply do not exist.

Contact with helping services, including primary care, is likely to have been lost, and homeless people are unlikely to be receiving treatment.

Specific problems

Major mental illness

The closure of long stay mental hospitals has not been responsible for the large number of homeless people who are mentally ill. Excessive rates of psychosis among homeless people have been reported since the 1950s. Few of the current homeless population have had long term hospital admissions, but most of those with psychiatric problems have had multiple brief admissions with poor follow up.

Shelter for many of these vulnerable people has been provided by hostels or reception centres. Although these institutions are supposed to provide only temporary accommodation, many people with chronic psychotic illnesses have lived in them for years. This may be because they are tolerant environments where, traditionally, little "rehabilitation pressure" is placed on residents. They have become de facto institutions, affording sanctuary but providing little adequate treatment and producing the same institutional deficits as did the old asylums.

Pathways to homelessness

- Unemployment
- Problem drinking among middle aged men
- Drug misuse among teenagers
- Lack of low rent housing
- Marital break up
- Clashes with family or friends
- Leaving local authority care
- Leaving the armed forces
- Leaving prison
- Episode of mental illness
- Children of homeless families

Very few people choose to have no home

Spectrum of housing needs

- People living in existing households in very unsatisfactory conditions
- Households sharing accommodation involuntarily
- Imminent release from institutional accommodation (prison, local authority)
- Insecure tenure (holiday letting, tied accommodation, mortgage default)
- Accommodation for homeless people (hostels, night shelters, bed and breakfast)
- No shelter ("roofless", "sleeping out" on streets or in parks or car parks)

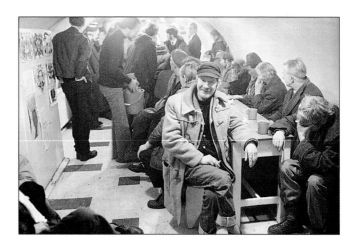

Figure 16.1. Many homeless people show signs of mental illness

Homelessness is often a consequence of severe mental illness

Anxiety and depression

Both anxiety and depression are common in homeless people. These may result from the stresses of living without a home, and they can be disabling, so trapping people in homelessness. Low level support is often all that is needed and can produce dramatic improvements. Referral for psychotherapy or counselling should be made as appropriate on clinical grounds.

Substance misuse

Alcohol has been the traditional substance of misuse for homeless men (women are less likely to have an alcohol problem), often having been the cause of homelessness in the first place. Hence the stigmatising stereotype that identifies all homeless people as alcoholics, despite the fact that in most British studies psychosis is at least as common as alcoholism. Alcohol accounts for the small but highly noticeable number of homeless people with severe cognitive problems.

Drug misuse is an increasing problem among the growing proportion of young homeless people. Opiate addiction has always been a minority problem, with the main drugs of misuse being amphetamines and benzodiazepines. The most common picture is of opportunistic misuse of multiple drugs, often with alcohol as well.

Dual diagnosis—Alcohol or drug misuse and psychosis are found increasingly in the same individual ("dual diagnosis"). Such patients are particularly difficult to help, not only because of the multiplying effect of the disruption caused by each problem, but also because they tend to fall between mainstream alcohol and psychiatric services.

Physical illness

Compared with the general population, homeless people suffer from considerably more untreated disease. Chronic chest, skin, and dental problems predominate and may exacerbate anxiety and depression.

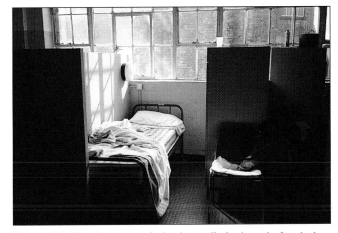

Figure 16.2. Hostel accommodation is usually basic and often lacks privacy. However, hostels may be tolerant and undemanding environments for homeless people with chronic mental illness

---

Physical disorders in homeless people

Offer to treat
- Chest infections
- Skin problems
- Other conditions amenable to a short course of treatment

Offer advice on
- Contraception
- Diet
- Smoking and alcohol consumption

Offer referral for
- Dental problems
- Alcohol and drug misuse

Barriers to care

Professional attitudes

Stereotyping—Health workers are not immune to the popular stereotypes that portray homeless people as being alcoholic, with personality disorder, feckless, and as having chosen their lifestyle. They often expect homeless patients to be both awkward and highly mobile: the myth of the "tramp".

"What difference can I make?"—Patients who are both homeless and mentally ill have a multiplicity of needs. Doctors' usual interventions assume the presence of the social factors (housing, adequate nutrition, and a social network) that made possible both health and treatment. Doctors may feel that they have nothing to offer when the absence of these factors seems to defeat any medical or psychiatric intervention.

Organisation of services

Communicaton—The multiple needs of homeless people who are mentally ill require help from several agencies—health, social, and housing—in addition to a specifically psychiatric input. This requires substantial communication between agencies, which, in spite of legislation on community care, is still the exception rather than the norm.

Psychiatric "No fixed abode" rotas—Many psychiatric units have a "No fixed abode" rota, which allocates homeless patients to a duty psychiatric team. Unless this also confers continuing responsibility for such patients, their care will be unnecessarily fragmented.

> **The difficulty in treating homeless people can produce a therapeutic nihilism that may not only prevent professionals from doing what they can but may even serve as a justification for neglect**

Desirable characteristics of a service for homeless people
- "Out there"
- Rapid response
- Informal
- Flexible
- Prepared to deal with a range of social as well as medical needs
- Collaborative, part of a wider service network
- Responsive to changing circumstances

Philosophies of care—Different agencies have differing philosophies of care: some operate non-interventionist policies that may prevent or delay referral. Most mental health services would consider that patients are unable to make informed choices when in the throes of a relapse of a severe mental illness. Many housing organisations take the view that people are always fully responsible for their choices and actions. This can lead to eviction if a disturbed or distressed patient is deemed, by his or her difficult behaviour, to have made a choice. To be fair, the inaccessibility of psychiatric help has often made it difficult for housing agencies to respond in any other way.

Homeless lifestyles

Priorities—Both physical and psychiatric care rank low in homeless people's list of priorities. The demands of securing immediate needs for survival—food, shelter, money—are more pressing than appointments with doctors or nurses.

Poor access to services—General practitioners are both gatekeepers and guides to most sources of psychiatric or psychological help. Homeless people with no regular general practitioner will often have to find their own way to these services, perhaps via an accident and emergency department. For obvious reasons, these departments are orientated towards brief intervention rather than continued involvement and advocacy.

Mobility—is as often forced on homeless people as it is chosen. Although much of this movement is relatively local, crossing the boundaries of catchment areas may lead to problems of both primary and secondary care services denying responsibility.

Alienation—Homeless people have often been disappointed by statutory services. Their predicament makes demands that these agencies cannot meet, often provoking inadequate or even punitive responses. Hospitals and general practitioners are reluctant to take them on, benefits regulations seem specially designed to penalise them, council housing departments are interested only in homeless families and the most vulnerable people, and the police may move them on or arrest them for drunkenness. It is not surprising that homeless people are often suspicious and distrustful of services that like to see themselves as caring and helping.

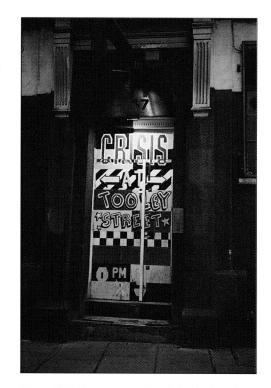

Figure 16.3. Entrance to a hostel for the homeless. Many homeless people use the same hostel—or a small number of hostels—on a regular basis. Thus, they may provide a reasonably reliable point of contact

Providing services

Improving access

Conventional clinic times will not do for homeless patients. It is more realistic to arrange meetings at times that fit in with their often irregular timetables. Even better is a drop-in service at a hostel or day centre where people can be seen quickly without appointment (Fig. 16.3).

Providing information

Voluntary agencies provide most of the social care and support for homeless people. These commonly include hostels, day centres, sources of cheap or free food and clothing, alcohol counselling services, and advice centres. Each health authority or hospital trust should obtain or create a directory that is concise enough to be of use in a busy ward, general practice, or accident and emergency department.

Referral

Referral to the local authority social services or housing department (homeless persons unit) may lead to a considerable improvement in a patient's accommodation but will often require the involvement of an advocate of some sort.

Providing homeless people with mental health services
- Initially, this may seem daunting, but it is relatively straightforward if it is a coordinated part of more general housing and social provision
- Don't do what you can't do, but make sure that you know someone who can
- Homeless people are rewarding to treat and grateful to those who treat them with respect

---

Useful addresses and voluntary organisations
Message Home
- A national freecall helpline for those who have left home or run away and wish to send a message
- Free helpline 0500 700 740

Shelter
- National Campaign for Homeless People, 88 Old Street, London EC1V 9HU
- Telephone 0171 505 2000

Finding a key worker or advocate—Treatment plans for homeless patients often fail because it is assumed that there is no carer with whom contact can be maintained. In fact, there is nearly always a person or organisation with whom they maintain contact and who should be informed. This might be a worker at a hostel or day centre, an alcohol counsellor, a minister of religion, a social worker, or a probation officer—the list is surprisingly long. Issues of confidentiality may arise, but these can be overcome by obtaining patients' written permission or by producing an edited, portable version of documents such as discharge summaries.

Treatment

Whatever the temptation to prescribe benzodiazepines for someone who is obviously distressed—don't do it. Although most homeless patients use their medication responsibly, it should not be forgotten that drugs such as the benzodiazepines, chlormethiazole, and procyclidine have a substantial and tempting street value.

Offer advice and treatment (including referral) for dental and other physical disorders.

Lack of supervision makes it unwise to attempt alcohol detoxification outside a well organised hostel sick bay, hospital, or alcohol unit. Paradoxically, hostels for the homeless can be good places to prescribe antipsychotic drugs. Since there is often little pressure to achieve quick results, it is possible to start with low doses and increase slowly. This usually avoids troublesome side effects and so reduces resistance to treatment.

Compulsory admission under the Mental Health Act is occasionally necessary, usually to treat an acute psychotic episode in which a patient becomes suicidal, violent, or dangerous in other ways (such as setting fires). Prompt intervention and treatment may mean that a hostel is prepared to accept a patient back when he or she is discharged from hospital.

Maintaining continuity of care for homeless patients

- Obtain, or create, a directory of local services for homeless people
- Get to know the hostels that a patient uses—there may be several in a relatively small locality
- Get to know the hostel workers and other people with whom patients may keep in contact
- Be prepared to offer short term courses of treatment
- Use simple treatment regimens (single drugs, once daily doses)
- Allow for patients' mobility—prepare a brief case summary for patients to carry with them or to be sent on request to other agencies
- Be prepared to accept patients back into your care and to restart treatment
- Build up trust—be accessible, flexible, and sensitive to patients' priorities

> **Do not prescribe drugs that may be misused**

Further reading

Craig T, Bayliss F, Klein O, Manning P, Reader L. *The homeless mentally ill initiative.* London: Department of Health, 1995

Craig TKJ, Hodson S, Woodward S, Richardson S. *Off to a bad start. A longitudinal study of homeless young people in London.* London: Mental Health Foundation, 1996

Gill B, Meltzer H, Hinds K, Petticrew M. *OPCS surveys of psychiatric morbidity in Great Britain. Report 7: psychiatric morbidity among homeless people.* London: HMSO, 1996

Haig R, Hibbert G. Where and when to detoxify single homeless drinkers. *BMJ* 1990;301:848-9

Shiner P, Leddington S, "Sometimes it makes you frightened to go to hospital . . . they treat you like dirt." *Health Services Journal* 1991 Nov 7:21-3

Williams D, Avebury K, eds. *People who are homeless.* London: HMSO, 1995

Lawrenson F. Runaway children: whose problem? *BMJ* 1997;314:1064

17 Mental health and the law

Ann Barker

The law relating to medical practice in general, and mental health in particular, is complex. This article provides a summary of the laws applying in England and Wales. Certain mental disorders are the only medical conditions for which the law permits treatment without the consent of the patient, but this can be undertaken only in a hospital or registered nursing home.

Mental Health Act 1983

Most treatment of mental disorder is undertaken voluntarily, whether in the community or on an outpatient basis or during a hospital stay. Compulsory admission of a patient from the community must be for one or more legal reasons set out in the Mental Health Act. Admission for assessment or treatment of a patient with a mental disorder may be necessary for the patient's health, the patient's safety, protection of others, or all of these.

Section 2 of the act allows for compulsory admission for assessment (and subsequent treatment), while section 3 allows for compulsory treatment when the category of mental disorder is already determined. These sections require recommendations from two doctors, one of whom is "approved" under section 12 of the act and one—usually the patient's general practitioner—who should know the patient. An application for admission is usually made by an approved social worker, but in certain circumstances the patient's nearest relative may fulfil this role.

The legal categories of mental disorder are mental illness, psychopathic disorder, and mental impairment, and the mental disorder must be so severe as to warrant treatment in hospital rather than in the community. The definitions of psychopathic disorder and mental impairment include a disorder of behaviour. For section 3, both categories must be considered treatable before admission to hospital is warranted. An important role of the patient's social worker is to ensure that resorting to hospital treatment is made only when necessary.

Emergency admission

Sections 4 and 5 of the Mental Health Act permit emergency admissions. When there is "urgent necessity" one doctor, preferably with previous knowledge of the patient, and a social worker or the nearest relative may compel admission under section 4. It is good practice that use of this section be converted to section 2 by recourse to an approved doctor.

If the patient is already an inpatient—but not an outpatient or someone attending an accident and emergency department—he or she may be prevented from leaving hospital by one doctor under section 5(2). If the doctor in charge of treatment is not a psychiatrist (for example, an obstetrician), he or she must act in person (not by proxy) and make immediate contact with a psychiatrist. A patient receiving treatment for both physical and mental conditions should be detained by the consultant psychiatrist or his or her nominated deputy.

Treating detained patients

In an emergency, treatment can be given under common law in the best interests of the patient. Only longer periods of detention, which involve assessment by two doctors, allow for

---

Legal pathways to compulsory treatment or care
Mental Health Act 1983

Section 2, 3 or 4—Admission to hospital from the community
Section 5—Detained by a nurse or a doctor while already an inpatient
Section 35, 36, 37, 38, or 41—Admission on the authority of a court after an offence
Section 47 or 48—Admission from prison on Home Office authority
Section 135—Taken by police from a private dwelling under a magistrate's warrant
Section 136—Taken by police from a public place to a place of safety

National Assistance Act 1948
Removal to suitable premises of people in need of care and attention

Powers of Criminal Courts Act 1973
Treatment as a condition of a probation order

Legal authority exists for supervision in the community but not for compulsory treatment (including drug treatment)

Legal categories of mental disorder

Mental illness—Not specified
Psychopathic disorder—A persistent disorder of mind (not specified) resulting in abnormally aggressive or seriously irresponsible conduct
Mental impairment and severe mental impairment—Arrested or incomplete development of mind with considerable or severe impairment of intelligence and impaired social functioning and abnormally aggressive or seriously irresponsible conduct

---

General guide to arranging compulsory admission from the community (local arrangements may vary)

Agencies involved
- General practitioner (or other doctor with prior knowledge of the patient)
- Doctor approved under section 12 (consultant psychiatrists for catchment area, doctors from local community mental health centre, or "on call" psychiatrist)
- Social worker approved under the act

Coordination
- The agency coordinating the assessment is usually decided by local agreement
- Involves arranging a time and place for the assessment, identifying a hospital bed, supplying legal documents (section papers), and arranging transport (such as an ambulance) and escort (doctor, community nurse, social worker, or police)

Urgency
- Attempt to judge the urgency of the situation in terms of safety and wellbeing of the patient and other people
- In emergency consider admission under section 4

Access (if patient will not grant access or submit to assessment)
- Try persuasion—Patient's general practitioner, community psychiatric nurse, relatives, or close friends may be able to persuade the patient
- In exceptional cases the social worker may apply to a magistrate for a warrant to force entry under section 135

Safety
- Do not act alone—Consider safety of the patient, staff, and others
- Should the police be asked to attend?
- Allow plenty of time—Most patients can be persuaded to cooperate if given enough time

medical treatment for mental disorder to be administered forcibly. However, electroconvulsive therapy may not be given to detained patients without their consent unless permission is obtained from the Mental Health Act Commission.

A detained patient's consent to psychiatric treatment must be reviewed after three months, and, if he or she does not consent, permission to continue treatment must be sought from a "second opinion approved doctor" appointed by the Mental Health Act Commission.

Treatment after a criminal oence

Of the six million criminal offences notified to the police each year, the vast majority are minor property offences, such as shoplifting, and are dealt with in magistrates' courts. Some 100 000 serious offences (such as homicide, grevious bodily harm, arson, and rape) proceed to the Crown Court.

Hospital orders—Either court may pass a hospital order under section 37 of the Mental Health Act for inpatient treatment when there is evidence of mental disorder, but only the Crown Court may make a hospital order under section 41, which allows the Home Office to place restrictions on a patient's movements. Patients under this order may be recalled to hospital if, for example, they do not take their medication in the community.

Probation orders—Outpatient treatment may be undertaken under a probation order with a condition of psychiatric treatment, provided that the patient agrees. Probation officers fulfil the role of social worker, and, in the event of a patient not complying with the conditions, he or she may be returned to court for an alternative sanction.

National Assistance Act 1948

Section 47 of this act allows for patients to be removed from their dwelling place to suitable premises, most often hospital, if they fulfil all the following conditions:
- They are living in insanitary conditions
- They are suffering from serious chronic disease or are aged or infirm or are physically incapacitated
- They are not receiving proper care and attention.

The doctor—usually a public health physician—makes a report to this effect, which then requires approval from the local court.

Consent to treatment

All treatment proposed by a doctor must be in the best interests of the patient. It is, however, a patient's right to give or withhold consent to examination or treatment. Procedures undertaken without consent can (though rarely) lead to an action for damages or a criminal prosecution for assault.

Consent may be implied, such as when a patient offers an arm for venepuncture, or expressed in oral or written form. Written consent is often necessary, but it is the explanation by the doctor that is paramount. Over the age of 16, only the patient can legally give consent, but the agreement of a close relative is sensible when it is impossible to gain consent from the patient.

When treatment for a physical disorder is necessary and the patient seems mentally disordered, a psychiatrist should be consulted to confirm the presence of mental disorder and the treatment of the medical condition be undertaken in the best interests of the patient. Mental incapacity includes dementia and mental handicap and may include other mental disorders. No one can give consent on behalf of these patients, but it is wise to seek the views of close relatives and to take a second consultant opinion. For irreversible procedures (such as

Welfare of detained patients
The rights of detained patients are overseen by two separate bodies, the Mental Health Review Tribunals and the Mental Health Act Commission

Mental Health Act Commission
- Oversees the welfare of patients detained in hospital and publishes a *Code of Practice* for their treatment, the authority of which is analogous to that of the *Highway Code* for motorists
Address—Maid Marian House, 56 Houndsgate, Nottingham NG1 6BG
Telephone 0115 950 4040.

Mental Health Review Tribunals
- Have the legal authority to release a patient from hospital if they consider that his or her mental disorder is not sufficiently severe, or that the risk to his or her own health or safety or the safety of others is not sufficiently great, to justify continued detention
- All patients detained in hospital for longer than 72 hours have the right to a tribunal hearing to argue the legality of their detention, and also the right to be legally represented at the hearing (including legal aid)
- There are three regional tribunals in England and one in Wales

---

Detention and treatment for the protection of others
- A "tiered" approach may be necessary for assessing the risk of harm to others: first dealing with immediate issues of safety and security and then assessing the continuing risks
- Risk implies uncertainty, and an attempt at accuracy requires great attention to detail
- It is important to assess the amount and type of harm predicted and the likelihood of this harm occurring, from "no risk" to "very high risk"

How much information do you have?
- As much information as possible should be sought from, for example, relatives, neighbours, probation officers, and even local newspaper reports

What kind of danger do you anticipate?
- Is it is likely that the patient will steal from shops, hit his or her partner, or take a knife and stab a stranger in the street?

How likely is it to happen?
- Where and under what circumstances is it likely that dangerous behaviour will occur?
- Does the patient always carry a knife, meet the potential victim every day at work, at football matches, or only at Christmas?

What could change to alter the risk?
- Dangerousness is never static but is a dynamic state that varies with mental health and variations in daily circumstances

Some predictors of danger to others
- History of violence or sexual assaults
- Misuse of alcohol or drugs
- Stops medication for major mental illness
- Young, male
- "Feels out of control"

Suicide by mentally disordered patients is much more common than homicide, but patients should be asked as routinely about thoughts of harming others as they are asked about suicidal thoughts

---

> **Mentally disordered patients can be capable of consenting to treatments, both for their mental disorder and for physical disorders**

The best interests of the patient
This is treatment that is
- Accepted by a responsible body of medical opinion
- Designed to save life, ensure improvement, or prevent deterioration of physical or mental health

sterilisation or amputation) permission should be sought from the Family Division of the High Court. Unconscious patients are incapable of giving consent and should be treated for life threatening disorders unless there is prior expressed evidence that the patient did not wish the treatment.

Children aged under 16 years who are able to understand their suggested treatment may give valid consent that cannot be reversed by their patients. If a child refuses the treatment it may still go ahead if the parents consent. For a child subject to a care order, the opinion of the local authority overrides parental consent. The doctor's paramount duty is to treat the child, and refusal by the parents should be noted in the clinical record. Girls aged under 16 may be provided with contraceptive advice or termination of pregnancy without parental consent if they forbid the doctor to seek it and the treatment is in their best interests.

Patients may give restricted consent (for example, Jehovah's Witnesses' refusal to permit blood transfusions), and a note should be made of the precise restriction made. A patient's choice of treatment may be overruled by an application to the Family Division of the High Court. A doctor can refuse to treat only if there is another doctor available to undertake treatment or if no harm will ensue.

Confidentiality

All members of a healthcare team should be aware of the duty of confidentiality, and case notes should be kept secured. A breach of professional confidentiality is viewed seriously by the General Medical Council. Information may be divulged with the patient's consent, preferably in writing, or on instruction from his or her solicitor who is assumed to convey that consent. After a patient's death, permission should be sought from the executor of his or her estate.

Difficulty commonly arises when a patient is in breach of the law. Wherever possible the doctor should attempt to gain the patient's consent to give information, or obtain a request from the court to submit a report. The doctor may breach confidentiality on the grounds of public interest if "the failure to disclose appropriate information would expose the patient, or someone else, to a risk of death or serious harm" but should be able to justify the decision. If in doubt, the doctor should consult his or her defence society.

Access to Health Records Act 1990

A health record relates to the physical or mental health of a patient, written by almost any professional except a social worker or teacher. Patients may read, have a copy, and have an explanation of their record. They may also apply to have their record corrected if they consider it inaccurate: in response, a correction may be made or the objection noted. Records made before 1 November 1991 are accessible only if necessary to make the later record intelligible.

Information about psychiatic patients is commonly given in confidence by relatives or carers, and divulging this information may put them at risk from the patient. In such cases parts of the medical record may be withheld from the patient.

> A valid consent to treatment requires a full explanation in non-technical language of the nature and purpose of the procedure to a patient capable of understanding the explanation and such explanation of the material risks that is reasonable in the circumstances by an appropriately qualified clinician for the particular procedure proposed on an ongoing basis without unfair or undue pressure

---

Difficulties in gaining consent
- Mental disorder
- Mental incapacity
- Children
- Restricted consent

> "I will respect the secrets which are confided in me, even after the patient has died"
> **Declaration of Geneva 1947**

Grounds for breaching patient confidentiality
Legal duty to release information
- Certain infectious diseases
- Registration of births and deaths
- Children at risk
- Prevention of terrorism
- Misuse of illegal drugs
- Termination of pregnancy
- Adverse reaction to drugs

Duty to comply with a request for information
- Report to a judge or chairman of a court
- Report to a coroner
- Release of medical record to police on order of a circuit judge
- Name and address to police in a road traffic offence

Access to medical records
A patient's request for access to his or her medical records should be respected Access may be restricted, or some information withheld, if
- The information is likely to cause serious harm to the mental or physical health of the patient
- The information is likely to cause serious harm to the mental or physical health of another person (not including health professionals)
- The information is about, or provided by, another individual (again not a health professional)

Further reading
Managing self-harm: the legal issues. *Drug Ther Bull* 1997;35:41–3

British Medical Association. *Rights and responsibilities of doctors.* 2nd ed. London: BMJ Publishing Group, 1992

British Medical Association, the Law Society. *Assessment of mental capacity: guidance for doctors and lawyers.* London: BMA, 1995

Davies T. Consent to treatment. *Psychiatr Bull* 1997;21:200–1

Department of Health, Welsh Office. *Code of practice. Mental health act 1983.* London: HMSO, 1993

Jones R. *Mental health act manual.* 5th ed. London: Sweet and Maxwell, 1996

18 Psychotropic drug treatments

Soumitra R Pathare, Carol Paton

This chapter takes a broad view of the factors affecting the choice and effectiveness of common drugs in psychiatric use. Specific treatment issues are dealt with in earlier articles in this book.

Antidepressant drugs

All antidepressants are equally effective in treating depression, and no single drug has been shown to have a more rapid onset of action than another. The choice of antidepressant is dictated by a combination of factors including the clinical presentation, the patient's physical health, the anticipated side effect profile, and the prescriber's preferences.

Types of depression—Certain types of depression respond better to particular classes of drugs, such as atypical depressive illness to monoamine oxidase inhibitors or mixed anxiety and depression to selective serotonin reuptake inhibitors. Patients with agitated depression respond well to a sedating tricyclic drug such as amitriptyline. If social withdrawal is prominent, a "stimulating" antidepressant such as imipramine or a selective serotonin reuptake inhibitor such as fluoxetine may help.

Suicide risk—Overall, selective serotonin reuptake inhibitors are safer than tricyclics in overdose, with dothiepin having been found to be the most toxic. Since suicide risk in any given patient is extremely difficult to predict, it has been argued that selective serotonin reuptake inhibitors should be the first choice of treatment in all cases of depressive illness. The financial implications of completely abandoning tricyclics in favour of selective serotonin reuptake inhibitors are enormous. However, the cost of drug related morbidity and treatment failure due to poor compliance must also be considered. For the moment, the most effective and economical way to prevent suicide is to
- Identify those at greatest risk of suicide
- Give small supplies to patients at risk—a week's prescription at a time
- Use a therapeutic dose of any antidepressant, not a small dose of a "safe" one. In the case of tricyclics this should be at least 150 mg/day.

Psychotic depression—The presence of delusions in depressive illness usually predicts a poor response to antidepressants alone. Addition of an antipsychotic drug will greatly improve the outcome. Trifluoperazine 5–10 mg daily is a reasonable choice in a healthy adult.

Dose and duration of antidepressant treatment

Many depressed patients are given too small a dose of antidepressant for too short a time, leading to poor response, repeated relapses, and increased morbidity. About 70% of patients respond to the first antidepressant administered if it is given at a therapeutic dose (such as amitriptyline 150 mg/day or fluoxetine 20 mg/day) for an adequate period (6–8 weeks).

If there is no response, and compliance is not in doubt, the dose should be increased if tolerated or the antidepressant changed to one from a different class. A further 10–15% of patients will respond to an alternative drug. If the response is still inadequate specialist referral is appropriate (Fig. 18.1).

For a single episode of depression, treatment should be continued after remission of symptoms for at least six months in younger patients and at least two years in elderly patients. If there are recurrent episodes then a maintenance dose of

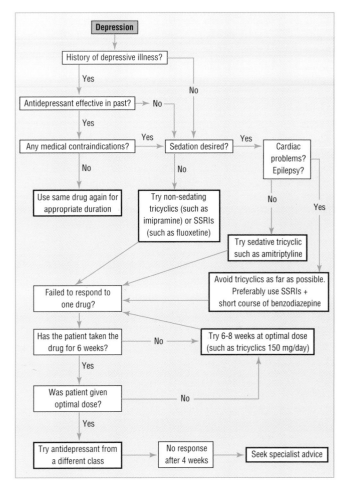

Figure 18.1. Decision tree for drug treatment of depression

Disadvantages of different classes of antidepressant
Tricyclic antidepressants
- Prominent anticholinergic side effects such as dry mouth, blurred vision, constipation, postural hypotension, and urinary retention
- Need to start with a small dose and increase gradually
- Weight gain is a substantial problem
- More serious side effects include
  Cardiac arrhythmias
  Seizures
  Depression of central nervous system (potentiated by alcohol)
- Toxic in overdose to varying degrees

Selective serotonin reuptake inhibitors
- Cost
- Development of serotonergic syndrome, characterised by headaches, gastrointestinal upsets, nausea, and anxiety
- Lack of sedation
- Potential for interactions with other drugs (warfarin, phenytoin, etc)
- Some distressing side effects (especially sexual dysfunction)

Monoamine oxidase inhibitors
- Main drawback is their dangerous interaction with tyramine rich foods and sympathomimetic drugs, which can lead to hypertensive crisis
- Anticholinergic side effects and hepatotoxicity
- Need for washout period

antidepressant or lithium should be considered for a much longer time. The importance of compliance should be emphasised, along with the risk of relapse if treatment is stopped prematurely: 65% of patients who stop treatment relapse within a year, compared with 15% of those who continue drug treatment.

Antipsychotic drugs

As with the antidepressants, no individual antipsychotic drug, except for clozapine, has been shown to be any more effective than another. All are effective in treating hallucinations, delusions, and thought disorder. Traditional antipsychotics have limited efficacy against the negative symptoms of schizophrenia, and the newer drugs (clozapine, olanzapine, risperidone, and sertindole) have some advantages in this respect.

The older, traditional compounds are usually differentiated by the degree of sedation they produce, with chlorpromazine being the most sedative and trifluoperazine the least (Fig. 18.2). The converse tends to be true for antipsychotic potency, with the more sedative drugs being less potent than their non-sedative alternatives. The high potency compounds are used primarily for treating acutely psychotic adults, while the low potency compounds are used when agitation is prominent or their sedative effects are desirable.

In elderly patients high potency compounds can produce severe extrapyramidal side effects while low potency drugs can lead to troublesome postural hypotension. All of these drugs are associated with increased morbidity in elderly people because of their adverse effects on mobility.

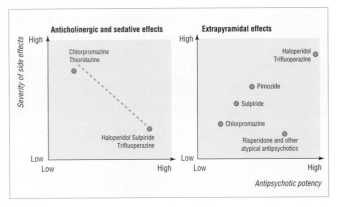

Figure 18.2. Relation between antipsychotic potency and severity of side effects

Response to antipsychotic treatment

Antipsychotics have a general calming effect and are useful in reducing arousal in the first few days of treatment (Fig. 18.3). The antipsychotic effect is more variable in onset, though as a general rule it is unusual to see much improvement before a week and most of the therapeutic gain tends to build up during the first six weeks. A therapeutic dose for an adequate period of time (such as haloperidol 10 mg/day for six weeks) will produce a good response in a third of patients, a partial response in a further third, and minimal or no response in the rest.

Dose of antipsychotic drugs

There is no evidence that high doses lead to a more rapid response or to improved efficacy in most patients who receive them. They lead to a high incidence of side effects and may be associated with sudden cardiac death. The Royal College of Psychiatrists' consensus statement on the use of high dose antipsychotics urges careful consideration and documentation

Side effects of traditional antipsychotic drugs

Common side effects	Rare side effects
● Sedation	● Epileptic seizures
● Anticholinergic effects—Made worse by antimuscarinic drugs (such as procyclidine)	● Bone marrow suppression
● Weight gain	● Abnormalities in cardiac conduction
● Extrapyramidal side effects	● Associated with unexplained sudden death
● Sexual dysfunction	
● Amenorrhoea	
● Photosensitivity (mainly chlorpromazine)	

Clozapine

- Recommended for treatment resistant schizophrenia; 60% of patients respond
- Treatment must be initiated by a consultant psychiatrist; may be prescribed by a general practitioner via shared care arrangement
- Lacks extrapyramidal side effects
- Main side effects—Sedation, hypersalivation, seizures
- 3% incidence of neutropenia, hence need for full blood count:
  Weekly for 18 weeks *then*
  Fortnightly until 52 weeks *then*
  Monthly if patient haematologically stable
- Avoid other drugs with myelosuppressive potential, such as depot antipsychotics, sulphonamides, chloramphenicol, cytotoxic drugs

Neuroleptic malignant syndrome

A rare but life threatening condition that can occur with any antipsychotic drug, irrespective of dose. Prompt identification is vital as patient needs specialist intensive medical treatment. It is most common when starting treatment or increasing the dose

Presentation
- Fever
- Muscular rigidity
- Confusion and impaired consciousness
- Autonomic instability (excessive sweating, labile blood pressure, tachycardia)
- Grossly raised serum creatinine kinase

Management
- Stop antipsychotic drugs immediately
- Manage psychotic disturbance with benzodiazepines or other sedatives
- Monitor cardiovascular and renal function
- After recovery from acute syndrome, consider cautiously reinstating antipsychotic drugs

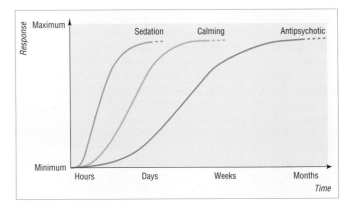

Figure 18.3. Relative times to achieve maximal effects of antipsychotic drugs

of all the relevant facts before embarking on the cautious use of high dose or regimens of multiple antipsychotics.

The conventional duration of treatment for a first episode of schizophrenia is one to two years after complete remission of symptoms. For repeated episodes, it is recommended that treatment is continued for at least five years and in some instances for life (Fig. 18.4).

Combination antipsychotics

Combinations of antipsychotic drugs should not generally be used as there is no evidence that this practice reduces side effects. The associated risks are not quantified. Exceptions to this rule include patients who are stabilised with depot preparations and require extra drug treatment during times of crisis and those who are changing from one antipsychotic to another. Combinations are occasionally used in treatment resistant schizophrenia, but this is usually dealt with by specialist units.

Anti-anxiety drugs

Mild anxiety is best treated by non-drug means such as training in anxiety management or relaxation techniques. Moderate to severe anxiety may benefit from a combination of these techniques and drug treatment in the form of antidepressants or very low dose antipsychotics. Benzodiazepines can be useful in treating acute anxiety, but tolerance to their effects can develop within days to weeks and they have a high potential for producing dependence.

The presence of anxiety is not necessarily an indication for the use of benzodiazepines. Non-selective β blockers such as propranolol have a role in treating physiological manifestations of moderate to severe anxiety and can be useful when these are prominent. If anxiety is part of an underlying depressive disorder an antidepressant is the only drug required, although a few days "cover" with a benzodiazepine may assist its introduction.

Similarly, insomnia is not a sufficient indication for the use of these drugs. Disturbed sleep is a common presenting problem in depression and alcohol misuse, so it is important to identify and treat the cause. Insomnia after a life event such as bereavement, or associated with extraneous factors such as noise and shift work, is also common. Many patients with a severe physical illness and pain complain of poor sleep. In all such cases, a short course of hypnotics should be prescribed only if the sleep disturbance is very severe, disabling, and causing extreme distress. Hypnotics started during a brief hospital admission should be stopped on discharge.

Anticholinergic drugs

Anticholinergic (strictly, antimuscarinic) drugs are used to relieve the extrapyramidal side effects of antipsychotic drugs. It is debatable whether anticholinergics should be given routinely when starting treatment with antipsychotic drugs. Extrapyramidal side effects can be frightening, and many patients refuse further antipsychotic drugs as a result. Prophylactic use of anticholinergics can prevent such occurrences and improve long term adherence to treatment.

However, anticholinergic drugs produce a pleasurable "buzz," which encourages misuse and dependence. Other side effects include drowsiness, dry mouth, blurred vision, and constipation. In elderly patients they can sometimes lead to an acute confusional state. They also interfere with the treatment of glaucoma and cause acute urinary retention in patients with prostatic hypertrophy. Hence, for most patients, anticholinergics should be prescribed only in the presence of obvious extrapyramidal side effects.

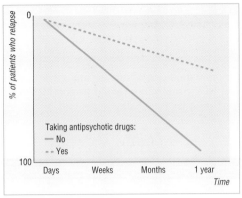

Figure 18.4. Effect of regular antipsychotic treatment on time to relapse

---

Side effects of benzodiazepines

- Daytime drowsiness
- Impaired memory and concentration
- Impaired reaction times—Patients should be warned of dangers of driving or operating machinery
- Potentiates depressive effects of alcohol on central nervous system—Can lead to accidental overdose
- Respiratory depression, especially in elderly patients and those with chronic airway disease
- Abrupt discontinuation can precipitate epileptic seizures
- Rarely, psychosis may occur during withdrawal

Prescribing benzodiazepines

Do
- Identify the cause of anxiety and insomnia and treat appropriately
- Encourage patients to consider non-drug methods of treatment
- Reserve benzodiazepines for anxiety or insomnia that is severe and disabling
- Use the smallest effective dose
- Use a short acting benzodiazepine for insomnia
- Use long acting benzodiazepine for daytime relief of severe anxiety
- Warn patients about dangers of dependence

Do not
- Prescribe for more than two weeks
- Give "routine" or repeat prescriptions
- Prescribe to patients who are liable to dependence

Extrapyramidal side effects of antipsychotic drugs

Parkinsonian syndrome
Presentation—Mask-like face, tremor at rest, rigidity, shuffling gait, motor retardation
Differentiate from withdrawal and apathy of schizophrenia syndrome
Treatment—Anticholinergic drugs

Dystonias
Presentation—Dystonic movements primarily affecting face, neck, and tongue and, rarely, the trunk and limbs. Oculogyric crisis
Treatment—Anticholinergic drugs, by parenteral route if severe

Akathisia
Presentation—Motor restlessness described by patients as a constant urge to move and an inability to sit still
Differentiate from agitation of schizophrenia
Treatment—Poor response to anticholinergic drugs. Reduce dose of antipsychotic drug if possible. Small doses of benzodiazepine or propranolol or cyproheptadine may help (seek specialist advice)

Tardive dyskinesia
A late side effect, usually apparent after many years of drug treatment but can occur sooner. Not associated with any particular drug and not dose dependent. Increasing age and cumulative dose are risk factors
Presentation—Involuntary movements affecting the face and the limbs. Sucking, smacking of lips, choreoathetoid movements of tongue. Choreiform movements in limbs. Rarely affects truncal muscles
Treatment—Gradually reduce dose of antipsychotic drug. Consider replacing with an atypical antipsychotic

Mood stabilising drugs

Lithium

The decision to use mood stabilisers should be taken only after consideration of the individual risk factors for any given patient. As a general rule, prophylaxis should be considered if two episodes of mood disorder (one being hypomania) occurred within a 2 year period.

When used in bipolar illness, the risk of early relapse of hypomania after discontinuation of lithium is high (higher than that expected from the natural course of bipolar illness). For this reason, it is probably wise not to start treatment in bipolar illness unless it is intended to continue it for at least 3 years. Major psychiatric illness is associated with a 30 fold increase in the suicide rate. Maintenance treatment with lithium reduces mortality from suicide in bipolar disorder to the same level as that seen in the general population. There is no convincing evidence that mortality from other causes is increased.

Side-effects tend to be directly related to plasma levels of lithium and are infrequent at levels below 1 mmol/L. Although up to a third of patients on long term lithium therapy develop polyuria, proven morphological changes in the kidney are confined to the distal tubules and collecting ducts, and are reversible. Polyuria is not a reason for discontinuing lithium unless the patient finds it intolerable. Hypothyroidism can be a problem but is not a sufficient reason for discontinuing lithium, replacement therapy with thyroxine should be commenced.

Severe gastrointestinal disturbance, drowsiness, ataxia, and dysarthria are early signs of lithium toxicity. If in doubt, lithium should be discontinued until a serum level can be obtained.

Bouts of vomiting, diarrhoea or any form of dehydration will lead to sodium depletion and therefore to increased serum lithium levels. Similarly a salt free diet is contra-indicated. It is also wise to ensure that the patient is aware of the importance of maintaining an adequate fluid balance.

Carbamazepine

Although used primarily as an anticonvulsant, carbamazepine is an effective mood stabiliser which offers a useful alternative when response to lithium is inadequate or side effects intolerable. It is more effective than lithium in rapid cycling bipolar illness (4 or more episodes per year). Carbamazepine is associated with leucopenia, hyponatraemia and abnormal liver function tests. It is prudent to have baseline values for LFTs, FBC and U&Es available.

It is important to start treatment with low dose and gradually titrate upwards over a period of 2 to 3 weeks. 100–200 mg twice daily would be a reasonable starting dose, and 300 mg twice daily an average maintenance dose. Too high a starting dose will lead to problems with ataxia, drowsiness, and nausea.

Contrary to popular belief, a therapeutic serum level range does not exist for the psychiatric uses of carbamazepine. Serum level monitoring therefore serves little purpose except to check compliance or suspected toxicity.

Carbamazepine is a hepatic enzyme inducer, increasing its own metabolism as well as that of several other commonly prescribed drugs for example, oestrogen containing oral contraceptives can be rendered ineffective. If these are used concurrently, preparations containing at least 50 mcg oestrogen are necessary. Conversely, hepatic enzyme inhibiting drugs can raise carbamazepine serum levels and so precipitate signs of toxicity. Erythromycin, cimetidine, calcium channel blocking drugs and dextropropoxyphene are commonly prescribed examples.

Starting and monitoring lithium

Preliminary tests (before starting treatment)
- Renal function tests (RFT)
- Thyroid function tests (TFT)
- Full blood count (FBC)
- Blood pressure
- ECG

Starting treatment
- Starting dose of 400 mg/day
- Do blood level after 7 days
- Titrate oral dose to achieve blood level of 0·4–1·0 mmol/L
- Monitor blood levels weekly until stable

Monitoring treatment
- Blood sample should be collected 12 hours after last dose
- If on twice daily regime, collect blood before morning dose
- Blood levels of lithium, TFT, RFT, FBC and ECG repeated every 3 months during maintenance phase

Improving compliance

Aim to increase patient's
- Comprehension
- Comfort
- Collaboration

The patient should feel more in control and less coerced

Strategies to improve compliance with drug treatment

- When starting treatment, explain the time course of effects. Patients need to be aware that any therapeutic effect will take weeks while side effects will be noticeable immediately. This should be emphasised again at follow up appointments
- Identify and treat side effects promptly. Prophylactic antiparkinsonian treatment is useful for some patients taking antipsychotic drugs
- Be realistic about what the drug can and cannot do. Many patients have highly unrealistic expectations of benefits
- When possible, start with a low dose and increase it gradually—this reduces the incidence of side effects
- Use minimum dose necessary to achieve desired therapeutic effects
- Use patient information leaflets to provide a written back up of oral information
- Involve patients in monitoring their own treatment

Depot antipsychotic preparations

- No additional efficacy over oral preparations
- Not recommended for use during the acute phase of an illness
- Not usually recommended after first episode of illness—Ideally, specialist opinion should be sought before starting depot treatment
- If patient has responded to an oral preparation of a particular drug, try a depot preparation of the same drug or another drug from the same class
- If reducing dose, gradual reduction (10% of dose at a time) is recommended
- Only useful in non-compliant patients if non-compliance is due to forgetting to take the oral drug or patient not keen to take tablets on a daily basis
- Of limited use with other causes of non-compliance, as patients can default on depot preparations as well

Compliance with treatment

Poor compliance, or adherence, with treatment is a major problem with almost all psychotropic drugs. Compared with patients who relapse in spite of good adherence, those with poor adherence to treatment are more severely ill at the point of readmission to hospital, have more frequent readmissions, are more likely to be admitted compulsorily, and have longer inpatient stays. Adherence itself has a protective effect distinct from the pharmacological benefits of the drug. Reasons for poor adherence involve problems with comprehension, comfort, and collaboration.

Comprehension—Problems include difficulties in appraising the importance of taking drugs. Patients and their families often have an inadequate understanding of the advantages and limitations of medication.

Comfort—This refers to unpleasant aspects of the treatment such as side effects. Patients with schizophrenia are highly likely to identify parkinsonian side effects as the reason for poor adherence, and non-adherers are less likely to have been prescribed antiparkinsonian medication. Dysphoria, sedation, weight gain, sexual disturbances, and galactorrhoea in female patients are other side effects of drugs that contribute to poor adherence. The side effects are usually experienced before any therapeutic effect, both with antipsychotic and antidepressant drugs.

Collaboration—Poor adherence can also be viewed as a result of a breakdown in the collaboration between patient and doctor. It has been argued that schizophrenic patients, particularly young people and those from ethnic minorities, perceive psychiatric treatment as coercive and disempowering. Promising results have been obtained with programmes that combine giving information with efforts to encourage schizophrenic patients to collaborate with professionals in monitoring their treatment.

Further information

- Contact your local hospital pharmacist who specialises in psychotropic medication
- In the United Kingdom and the Republic of Ireland, information may be obtained by telephoning regional drug information services or poisons information centres. An up to date list of telephone numbers is given in the current *British National Formulary*
- National Schizophrenia Fellowship (NSF) and the Royal College of Psychiatrists produce patient information leaflets which are clear and informative
- Clozaril Patient Monitoring Service (Sandoz Pharmaceuticals) provides information about all aspects of clozapine treatment to doctors who are registered with the service

Further reading

Long-term management of people with psychotic disorders in the community. *Drug Ther Bull* 1994;32:73–7

Three new antidepressants. *Drug Ther Bull* 1996;34:65–8

Bazire S. *Psychotropic drug directory*. Dinton, Wiltshire: Quay Books, 1995

Davies T. Consent to treatment. *Psychiatr Bull* 1997;21:200–1

National Medical Advisory Committee. *The management of anxiety and insomnia*. Edinburgh: HMSO, 1994

Symposium: prescribing for the psychiatric patient in the non-specialist setting. *Prescribers J* 1996;36:181–228

Thompson C. Consensus statement. The use of high-dose antipsychotic medication. *Br J Psychiatry* 1994;164:448–58

19 Psychological treatments

Phil Richardson

The range of procedures that pass for a psychological treatment is broad. Over 450 distinct forms of psychotherapy have been identified, although many can be reduced to a narrower set of therapy types. The great diversity of available psychological treatments remains a potential source of confusion for referrers, service users, and purchasers. Confusion may also surround standards of training and practice. Training in psychotherapy and counselling abounds in Britain, which has no formal registration for either activity and no single professional accreditation body.

The recent review of psychotherapy services in the NHS underlines the efficacy and importance of psychological treatments for mental disorders. A joint statement from the British Psychological Society and Royal College of Psychiatrists identifies the need to develop integrated psychological therapy services within the NHS that can offer assessment, treatment, and training in psychological treatments.

Referral to a coordinated psychological treatments service may obviate the need for general practitioners and others to make difficult referral decisions about particular forms of treatment. However coordinated treatment services are not yet widely available, and referrers may be left to find their way through a maze of local services.

Cognitive-behaviour therapy

The term cognitive-behaviour therapy refers to a group of therapies that include behaviour therapy, behaviour modification, and cognitive therapy in various combinations. Despite their theoretical distinctness, the dividing line between cognitive and behaviour therapies is a fine one.

Behavioural approaches draw on the principles of Pavlovian "classical" conditioning (systematic desensitisation, aversion therapy), Skinnerian operant conditioning (contingency management, activity scheduling), or social learning theory (participant modelling). A formal behavioural analysis of a patient's problem is typically followed by individually tailored application of techniques to change behaviour. A change in behaviour is viewed as paramount, both as therapeutic aim in its own right and in mediating other symptomatic improvement.

Cognitive approaches emphasise how cognitions mediate feelings and behaviour. They aim to modify thought processes directly. Therapy consists of identifying maladaptive and often automatic thought patterns (such as hopelessness in depression) and teaching patients to recognise and challenge these.

In fact, cognitive therapists commonly use behavioural techniques as a way of learning about cognitive responses to events (such as exposure to a frightening situation). Conversely behavioural work often focuses on cognitive activity (such as mental images of a feared object in desensitisation).

Psychodynamic therapy

Psychodynamic approaches aim to go beyond symptomatic change by resolving the unconscious conflicts that are thought to underlie symptoms. Long term psychodynamic psychotherapy may last several years and seeks to achieve a fundamental change in personality. Its availability in the NHS is limited: few services can offer it on an inpatient basis, though several retain some scope for outpatient work.

Psychological treatments most commonly available in NHS
- Cognitive-behaviour therapy
- Psychodynamic psychotherapy
- Family therapy
- Group therapy
- Various forms of counselling
- Eclectic and integrative approaches

Cognitive-behaviour therapy
Psychotherapies
- Based on both behavioural and cognitive theories
- Structured
- Prescriptive rather than primarily exploratory
- Uses formal techniques for behavioural or cognitive change
- Focused on enabling patients to think and act differently

Treatment
- Individual or group
- Short term or long term
- Inpatient or outpatient
- Typically, it is offered on an individual outpatient basis for a limited course (between 8 and 24 weekly therapy sessions)

Indications for cognitive-behaviour therapy*
Type of problem
- Marked anxiety (panic, phobias, post-traumatic stress disorder, generalised anxiety disorder)
- Obsessions and compulsions
- Depression (especially with negative thoughts about self and others)
- Behavioural problem (eating disorders, sleep problems, uncontrollable anger, habit disorder)

Severity of problem—Moderate to severe
Chronicity of problem—Six months or more
Patient factors—Preference for change in symptoms or other concrete or practical target rather than for self exploration

*Adapted from Cape et al (see reading list)

Psychodynamic psychotherapy
Psychotherapeutic techniques
- Exploratory
- Based on psychoanalytic theory, the distinctive feature of which is the focus on resolution of unconscious conflicts

Treatment
- Makes direct use of the transference (the patient's experience of the therapist and therapeutic relationship)
- Aims to promote greater conscious understanding of difficulties by the patient and to enable assimilation of potentially painful and previously avoided experience
- Traditionally long term, but brief variants also available

Brief psychotherapy typically lasts for six months with weekly or twice weekly sessions. Therapeutic work is focused on specific issues in the expectation that improved understanding will enable patients to arrive at more lasting symptomatic change through a process that may extend beyond the end of the treatment.

There has been a growing rapprochement in recent years between the perspectives of psychodynamic and cognitive therapists. For example, a number of psychoanalytic concepts have been recast within a cognitive framework, but the therapeutic focus on the resolution of unconscious conflict remains a distinctive feature.

Counselling

There is no universally agreed definition of counselling and limited consensus over the distinction between counselling and psychotherapy. In practice, counselling is commonly practised in primary care and the voluntary sector, usually on a short term basis (4–10 sessions) by individuals who are not from the core mental health professions but usually have a formal qualification in counselling itself.

A broad distinction can be made between methods based on a specific theoretical framework (such as psychodynamic counselling) or targeting a particular problem (as in bereavement counselling) and generic counselling, which draws on a range of general interpersonal skills (such as reflective listening) and, in Britain, is commonly built on a humanistic or client centred foundation. Counselling is often used to help people cope better with the distress associated with immediate crises, to understand better their reactions to events, and to make decisions more effectively about important issues.

Eclectic and integrative approaches

Many practitioners of psychological treatments draw on the principles of various therapeutic approaches while working with an individual patient. For example, clinical psychologists may develop a broad based psychological formulation of a patient's problem using general psychological principles. Depending on the identified foci for intervention, several different methods may then be combined in the course of treatment. This eclectic approach has the advantage of flexibility, but it is difficult to evaluate since its nature changes from case to case and therapist to therapist.

Integrative approaches to therapy also combine the precepts and practices of different therapeutic methods, but in a way that recombines the elements to form a new coherent structure. In Britain cognitive-analytic therapy is a promising and increasingly popular form of brief integrative therapy which builds on the elements of both cognitive-behaviour therapy and psychodynamic psychotherapy.

Family therapy

Traditional family therapy exemplifies the "systemic" approach to understanding and modifying problematic behaviour and experience. The family (or other social system), rather than the individual patient, becomes the focus of understanding and intervention. A patient's problem is seen as serving a strategic function in maintaining some aspect of the family's functioning. The therapist's task is to identify this function and help the family move towards a more adaptive mode of operation.

Family therapists may use direct behavioural modification of a symptom, not as a therapeutic end in itself but as a means to identify the dysfunctional family system. Modifying the system

---

Indications for psychodynamic psychotherapy*

Type of problem
- Personality problems and severe interpersonal difficulties
- Any symptomatic presentation in which the problem can be understood in terms of patient's life circumstances or way of viewing the world

Severity of problem—Moderate to severe

Chronicity of problem—One year or more

Patient factors
- Interest in self exploration
- Adequate capacity to tolerate frustration and psychic pain

*Adapted from Cape et al (see reading list)

Indications for counselling*

Problems
- Adjustment reactions (to life events, illness, loss, etc)
- Situational anxiety or stress
- Low mood or subclinical depression
- Marital or relationship problems
- Interpersonal problems

Severity of problem—Mild to moderate

Chronicity of problem—Recent onset (<1 year) except for interpersonal problems

Patient factors—Preference for brief treatment

*Adapted from Cape et al (see reading list)

Problems in evaluating the psychotherapies
- A relative shortage of controlled trials examining the efficacy of psychodynamic therapies
- Evidence which reaches the highest standards of methodological rigour (from well conducted randomised controlled trials) is least typical of ordinary clinical practice, where the conditions of the controlled trial are least likely to apply
- Treatment trials and reviews are commonly organised around problem domains (anxiety, depression, etc), and tell us about the progress of the average treated patient compared with that of the average untreated one. Evidence from research on the relation between patient characteristics and therapy outcome points to the fact that there is no average patient

---

Where to find help
- Self help groups and voluntary organisations are available in many areas and may provide counselling and assertiveness training as well as psychotherapy for specific psychological problems
- Local libraries often stock self help manuals, relaxation tapes and other helpful material as well as lists of local voluntary services
- Leaflet *Finding a therapist* is available from the British Confederation of Psychotherapists, 37 Mapesbury Road, London NW2 4HJ (0181 830 5173)
- A counsellor or psychologist, located in a primary care setting, will deal with a wide range of minor psychological problems and refer patients on to specialist services when appropriate
- Marital or couple therapy is available from RELATE, or other voluntary organisations, in many areas
- Patients with phobic and obsessional disorders may be referred for behavioural treatment
- Patients with anxiety or depression may be referred for cognitive-behaviour therapy or cognitive-analytic therapy (depending on local provision)
- Patients with longstanding "neurotic" or personality problems may benefit from referral for psychodynamic therapy

itself may also be achieved through the planned application of various specific technical manoeuvres (such as positive reframing of the symptom, symptom prescription, paradoxical injunction).

In principle, systemic approaches to therapy make no prior assumption about the membership of the social group at which the intervention is targeted. "Adult" families, partial families, and other social groups are equally eligible for systems-based work. Family therapy is often available in child and adolescent mental health services, where a child presents initially as the patient but is viewed as the vehicle of expression of a dysfunctional family system.

A similar approach might be considered in any case in which there is obvious family involvement in the presenting problem. There is evidence for the effectiveness of this approach in eating disorders (especially in younger anorectic patients), psychophysiological disorders, and disruptive disorders in childhood.

Group therapy

Group therapy is a portmanteau term for a wide range of therapeutic approaches in which several patients come together for therapy at the same time and place with one or more therapists. Therapeutic groups may be run according to the principles of any theoretical approach (for example, cognitive-behaviour therapy, psychodynamic therapy); they may be open (in which new members can join the group after its inception) or closed; inpatient or outpatient; time limited or open ended; and their focus may be highly specific (anxiety management groups) or very broad (psychoanalytic group psychotherapy).

Although the economic advantages of therapeutic groups are self evident, group therapy is not a collective or diluted form of individual therapy. Virtually all group therapies draw on the idea that group processes themselves may be therapeutic. Whenever individual psychotherapy is being considered then it may also be worth considering referral for group therapy. However, assessment for inclusion in a group must take account of the specific group's characteristics, and of the patient's preference for individual therapy or aversion to a group.

Choice of therapeutic method

Neither a psychiatric diagnosis nor a clearly identified psychological problem can be regarded as automatic pointers to a particular psychotherapy of choice. Choice of treatment requires assessment of factors that bear on the probable success of a particular treatment for a particular patient. When possible, initial referral should be to a coordinated psychological treatments service with expertise in assessment and access to a range of specific therapies, including specialist clinics (such as for psychosexual problems).

In principle, these decisions should be evidence based, but, as in several other areas of health care, the available evidence is largely insufficient to the task. Cape et al have collated the main empirical and consensus evidence of the benefits of the most common forms of individual psychological treatment available in Britain in the form of a referral guideline (see further reading list).

Family psychoeducation in schizophrenia
- In recent years a distinct form of family work has been developed for families of schizophrenic patients
- After the discovery of the critical importance for recovery—or relapse—of the family's responses to the patient after a schizophrenic episode, a form of family therapy has been developed using educational, behavioural, and skills training approaches to enable family members to interact in ways that reduce the likelihood of subsequent relapse
- There is good evidence for the effectiveness of these methods, and training in them is becoming increasingly available to psychologists, psychiatrists, and nurse therapists

---

Main organisations accrediting psychotherapists in Britain

United Kingdom Council for Psychotherapy (UKCP)—Accrediting body for professional training in psychotherapy, it lists 71 training organisations in its 1995–6 national register but does not include all organisations offering psychotherapy training
British Confederation of Psychotherapists (BCP)—Comprises 10 psychotherapy organisations and includes most consultant psychotherapists in the NHS
British Association for Counselling (BAC)—Accredits a large number of formal training courses in counselling
Royal College of Psychiatrists (RCPsych)—Provides specialist training guidelines and accreditation criteria for the psychological therapies
British Psychologial Society (BPS)—Provides specialist training guidelines and accreditation criteria for the psychological therapies
English National Board for Nursing (ENB)—Approves a network of specialist nurse therapy training courses

Members of other mental health professions (occupational therapists and art therapists) are increasingly likely to offer counselling or other psychological treatment methods

---

Factors affecting choice of psychotherapeutic method

The problem	The patient
● Nature	● Preferences
● Chronicity	● Interests (focused on symptoms or interested in self understanding)
● Severity	● Attitudes ("psychological mindedness")
● Complexity	● Capacities (to tolerate painful emotions in therapy)

Further reading

Burns D. *The feeling good handbook*. Harmondsworth: Penguin, 1990
Cape, J, Durrant K, Graham J, Patrick M, Rouse, A. *Counselling and psychological therapies: guideline and directory*. London: Camden and Islington Medical Audit Advisory Group, 1996
Davies, TW. Psychosocial factors and relapse of schizophrenia. *BMJ* 1994;309:353–4
Enright SJ. Cognitive behaviour therapy—clinical applications. *BMJ* 1997;314:1811–6
NHS Executive. *NHS psychotherapy services in England. Review of strategic policy*. Wetherby: Department of Health, 1996
Roth A, Fonagy P. *What works for whom? A critical review of psychotherapy research*. New York: Guilford, 1996
Royal College of Psychiatrists, British Psychological Society. *Psychological therapies for adults in the NHS*. London: Royal College of Psychiatrists, 1995 (Council Report CR37)
Smith ML, Glass GV, Miller TI. *The benefits of psychotherapy*. Baltimore: Johns Hopkins University Press, 1980

20 Risk management in mental health

Teifion Davies

Risks and uncertainties abound in all branches of medicine, and assessing risk has always been an important aspect of clinical work. This is not confined to psychiatry: any patient may, as a consequence of an illness or its treatment, be exposed to risk or pose a risk to other people.

However, a formal assessment of risks to patients (due to their illness or its treatment) or to other people (due to violence or neglect by a patient) is increasingly seen as a routine component of psychiatric management and part of a patient's care plan under the care programme approach. Previous chapters have dealt with the major risks associated with specific mental health problems. This chapter draws together the common features of clinical risk management in mental health.

General principles

Strictly, a risk is the probability of an event occurring, where the event may be desirable (such as recovery from illness) or undesirable (such as side effects of drug treatment, relapse, suicide, or harm to others). Risk management has three principal components: identification, analysis, and control.

Identification

The essential first stage, which may seem obvious, is recognising that risks may arise from all aspects of clinical work and provision of health care. Factors as diverse as the layout of a surgery or ward, staffing levels and training, design of documents and records, means of communication between services, and prescribing practices may raise or lower risks. These "background" factors apply to all patients and clinical situations, but the need to be aware of them extends well beyond the doctors and nurses in the front line.

The specific risks associated with particular clinical situations or groups of patients should be identified. This will include the type and frequency of risks, the circumstances in which they arise, and the people subjected to them. In any healthcare organisation (such as hospital or general practice surgery) identification will depend on well developed programmes of audit and quality assurance, the prevalent "culture" and attitudes, and available knowledge.

Analysis

Risk is an actuarial concept, and analysis depends on quantifying several variables—risk factors—and their interactions. While some risk factors (such as a patient's personality) may remain constant over long periods, the size of others will vary (for instance, with changes in mental state or environment). So the estimated probability of occurrence will vary with time, and range from zero (no chance of the event occurring) to one (complete certainty that the event will occur).

The tests used to quantify a particular risk will be subject to the same constraints of sensitivity and specificity, and of errors of estimation, that apply to any measurement technique.

Control

Control of risk depends on the type of risk identified, its estimated size, and the resources available. Formal programmes for risk management in healthcare organisations

---

Clinical risks and clinical decision making

- All clinical decisions carry risks, and decision making should be seen as part of risk management
- Decisions may concern type of diagnosis, choice of treatment, need for admission to hospital, or fitness for discharge from hospital. In mental health, decisions may also concern compulsory admission and treatment and safety of other people
- Decisions often involve a choice between several options, each of which has its associated risks
- Decisions may involve comparing different risks (treating a patient with antipsychotic drugs may cause severe side effects, while not treating the patient may risk violence to others)
- None of the available options may be clearly superior to all the others
- Whenever possible, options should be discussed in a multi-disciplinary context
- The reasons for choosing a particular option should be stated clearly in the care plan, including
  Which options were considered
  What information was available
  The perceived risks of each option
  What changes in circumstances would prompt a review of the decision

---

Identifying risks

Type—Suicide, self harm, aggression, behavioural disturbance, damage to property, violence
Setting—Hospital ward, outpatient clinic, general practice, home, community
Timescale—Immediate, short term, medium term, and long term
Risk factors—Demographic (population of patients), patient (specific)
Disorder—Depression, schizophrenia, personality disorder, dementia, phobic anxiety, panic disorder

---

Case history: Risk of violent behaviour associated with acute psychotic disorder

Mr C, a 22 year old student at a teacher training college, became increasingly withdrawn and isolated, spending several days alone in his room at a hall of residence. He consulted the student health physician with complaints that "something was going on" and his mind was being read by the students living on the floor above his room. He was prescribed antipsychotic drugs, and referred to the local psychiatric clinic. He stopped taking his drug treatment after two days because of unacceptable side effects, which he attributed to "being poisoned."

A week later, he set a fire in his room in the belief that the smoke would prevent his thoughts being read. Considerable damage was caused, but prompt action by the emergency services prevented loss of life. He was arrested and charged with arson with intent to endanger life. At psychiatric interview, he showed features of paranoid schizophrenia, and the court ordered that he should be detained for treatment under section 37 of the Mental Health Act.

He was treated with gradually increasing doses of antipsychotic drugs, and responded well with few side effects. He returned to his college course after one year, with the knowledge and support of the college authorities.

emphasise economic aspects: weighing the resources needed to control risks against the anticipated costs of untoward events. "Costs" include effects on staff morale and damage to the organisation's reputation as well as more obvious clinical and legal costs.

Staff should be aware of the likely risks in their sphere of practice and of the risk management strategies. Since risk implies uncertainty there should be a culture of "expecting the unexpected," and of knowing what to do if the unexpected occurs. This will include a rapid response to untoward events, caring for victims (patients, staff, and others), and recording information.

Recent inquiries have pointed to the need to warn potential victims of important risks, to take account of their fears, and plan for their safety.

Clinical risk

Clinical risk concerns the potential for harm posed by, or inflicted on, an individual patient. The risk of a clinically important event occurring is best regarded as ranging from low (very unlikely) to high (very likely). This restricted range of probabilities takes account of the difficulties in applying actuarial data derived from populations to individual clinical situations.

Clinical risk factors divide roughly into two types: demographic and patient factors. Demographic factors relate to the risks in populations of patients, and tend to be relatively fixed or slowly evolving in time; they comprise the baseline level of risk in that population, but have poor temporal resolution. Patient risk factors form a pattern that is specific to a particular patient: they may be highly variable in time, so their estimation improves the accuracy of prediction in the short term.

In mental health the risks of greatest concern are suicide, self harm, violence to others, and neglect of dependents. Other risks are those familiar in all branches of medicine: morbidity and cumulative disability from illness, side effects of medical treatment (such as drugs or electroconvulsive therapy), and untoward outcomes of other treatments (including psychotherapy).

Clinical risk assessment

The reliability or predictive value of a clinical risk assessment is greatest at the time it is performed and declines rapidly afterwards (Fig 20.1). For this reason, each risk should be dealt with separately, its timescale (immediate, short term, medium term, or long term) delineated, and a time set for a further assessment to be made. A full risk assessment will require attention to each of these time periods, and of their interplay with the patient's diagnosis and treatment.

Immediate risks—These require immediate action to avoid an untoward event. They may arise from a sudden crisis in a patient's life or from fluctuations in his or her mental state. Assessment should focus on the patient's observed behaviour, level of emotional arousal, expression of intentions or threats, and psychomotor agitation, supplemented by as full an examination of the mental state as practicable.

Short term risks are predictable over the next few hours or days. Assessing these requires a knowledge of the patient's insight, coping mechanisms, and level of support, as well as an evaluation of ongoing crises and their potential resolution.

Medium term risks are those expected during the current episode of illness. The patient's provisional diagnosis and likely adherence and expected response to treatment are important in predicting risks during the current episode. The presence of specific risk factors (such as depressive, persecutory, and emotional phenomena) should be allowed for in the care plan.

Practical steps in managing a patient's risk

Accumulate information from clinical and non-clinical sources—This should include the current mental state and response to treatment. Include eye witness accounts, and details from family and neighbours where necessary

Identify gaps and discrepancies in the history—Are there periods during which the patient lost contact with services? If so, attempt to obtain missing information

Construct a chronological listing of significant events in patient's life— Include episodes of violence or suicidal behaviour, episodes of illness, treatment and response

Identify patterns of behaviour—Is risk taking haphazard, associated with specific circumstances (such as relapse of illness, social upheavals, drug or alcohol misuse), or particular people (such as family, neighbours, passers-by in the street)?

Assess risk of similar events recurring—Will the patient be exposed to similar situations in the future? If so, what can be done to minimise risk of harm occurring?

Disseminate information to all involved in the patient's care—All members of the clinical team should be aware of signs of relapse, or of impending violent or suicidal behaviour. The general practitioner should be included at all stages of discussion

Discuss the risks with the patient and his or her carers—Outline the perceived risks and the care plan. Indicate clearly whom to contact in an emergency. Respect confidentiality, but avoid being drawn into collusion or "keeping secrets." Make it clear that, in the interests of safety, information should be shared on a "need to know" basis

Treat mental disorder—Always prescribe adequate drug treatment, and appropriate psychological interventions, as indicated. Where there is a risk that drugs will be misused, arrangements should be made for safe storage and administration

Keep clear clinical records—This will facilitate the task of future risk assessment

Review the risk assessment and care plan—The value of an isolated assessment diminishes rapidly, and depends on changes in a patient's mental state and circumstances. Reviews should be scheduled at regular intervals, and any important changes should trigger earlier review

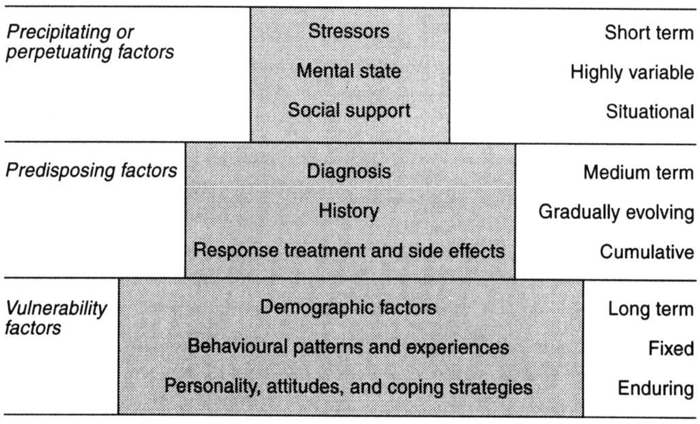

Precipitating or perpetuating factors	Stressors	Short term
	Mental state	Highly variable
	Social support	Situational
Predisposing factors	Diagnosis	Medium term
	History	Gradually evolving
	Response treatment and side effects	Cumulative
Vulnerability factors	Demographic factors	Long term
	Behavioural patterns and experiences	Fixed
	Personality, attitudes, and coping strategies	Enduring

Factors near the top of the hierarchy have greater temporal resolution in predicting immediate risks, while those lower down confer long term vulnerability. Factors at all levels contribute to a patient's response to his or her current circumstances

Figure 20.1 Risk factor hierarchy

Long term risks—These are the "baseline" risks that a patient exhibits between acute episodes of illness and which may remain reasonably constant or evolve gradually over many years. They are influenced by demographic factors such as the patient's age, sex, and social class. For a specific patient, these will be modified by diagnosis, enduring personality factors (such as emotional instability, poor coping, and low tolerance of frustration), social circumstances, and patterns of behaviour (such as remorse, help seeking, alcohol and drug misuse, and adherence to treatment).

Sources of information

In assessments of immediate and short term risks, the patient's observed behaviour and his or her mental state provide most information. In order to assess longer term risks and place short term risks in context, as much collateral information as possible should be sought. This will include general practice records and medical and psychiatric case notes, and may require tracing contacts with services in other districts. In some cases police or probation service records and local newspaper reports may provide further information.

Personal accounts from family, friends, neighbours, or healthcare staff may be particularly important for providing details of unrecorded incidents of dangerous or self harming behaviour. It is worth remembering that these people may be the ones most at risk from a potentially violent patient.

Interviews, handled sensitively, may serve the dual purpose of gaining information and informing potential victims of risks and contingency plans.

In practice, it is easiest to build up a picture of the risks posed by an individual patient if the clinical case notes provide a simple chronological record. It is important to remember that the structure of case notes should always be subservient to the function of clinical risk management.

Suicide

Death by suicide is about three times as common in men as women at all ages: the risk rises steeply in old age. In recent years the rate in young, often unemployed, men has risen by about 75%, and some surveys have noted similar increases in women. Several demographic factors are associated with raised risk of suicide, but these have poor sensitivity and specificity when applied to individuals. This may be because of the clear interaction between such factors as young age, unemployment, social deprivation, and alcohol and drug misuse.

Several mental disorders carry a high risk of suicide, the most important being depression (about 30 times the risk in the general population), schizophrenia, and alcohol dependence. However, "neurotic" disorders (such as social phobia and panic attacks) and personality disorders (particularly those with emotional instability or self harm) also confer an increased risk.

Assessment

In assessing an individual patient's suicide risk, careful evaluation of depressive symptoms (such as hopelessness)—together with direct inquiry about suicidal thoughts, intentions, and plans—is most important. Other critical factors are the nature of the precipitating events, the presence of serious physical illness, and the presence of social support (especially personal relationships).

Risks to others, especially dependent or physically ill relatives, should be considered. A patient experiencing nihilistic ideas or overwhelmed by a relative's chronic illness may contrive a "suicide pact" or mercy killing as part of his or her own suicide plans.

Case history: Risk of violent behaviour associated with social phobia

Miss B, a 30 year old woman with a history of social phobia became agitated while standing in the checkout queue of a busy supermarket. Her behaviour roused the suspicions of the store detective, who instructed two security guards to block the exit to the store. Her desire to escape became intolerable, and she struck a 10 year old girl who was standing in front of her in the queue.

She was arrested, but became aggressive and unmanageable when placed in a police van with four police officers. She was taken in handcuffs to the local hospital for assessment, and required tranquillisation to prevent her assaulting staff.

At interview, a clear history was elicited of social phobia associated with intolerable feelings of being trapped. She had no formal forensic history, but recalled damaging a telephone box several years earlier when she felt trapped inside.

Case history: Risk of violent behaviour in a "medical" patient

Mr A, a 56 year old married man with a long history of diabetes mellitus, was admitted to a medical ward of the general hospital for investigation of chest pain. He had no history of psychiatric disorder. As his meal was served, he became distressed with incoherent speech, and threw his plate at a nurse. He lost consciousness and collapsed.

Urgent tests showed no cardiac abnormality, but his blood glucose concentration was < 1.0 mmol/l. After correction of hypoglycaemia, he recovered consciousness with no recall of the events preceding his collapse. Enquiry revealed that he had behaved similarly on several previous occasions, at home and at work, but the incidents had been regarded as trivial and not recorded.

Demographic factors associated with high risk of suicide
- Male
- Age over 40 (but also increasingly in young men)
- Social class V
- Unmarried or socially isolated
- Family disruption (such as bereavement or divorce)
- Social disruption (loss of home, unemployment, redundancy, retirement)
- Family history of mood disorder or suicide
- Some occupations–farmers, doctors
- Mental disorder–especially depression, schizophrenia or alcohol dependence
- Personality disorder–especially young men with history of self harm, drug or alcohol misuse
- Physical illness–especially chronic, painful
- Previous suicide attempts or episodes of deliberate self harm

Patient factors associated with high risk of suicide
- Depression–including the depressed phase of bipolar affective disorder
- Schizophrenia–especially young men, with depressive symptoms, recurrent relapses, fear of deterioration, prominent side effects from drug treatment
- Anxiety disorders–especially associated with social phobia and panic attacks
- Recent life events–especially when lacking social supports or relationships
- Preparations–hoarding tablets, saying goodbyes, putting personal affairs in order
- Mental state–guilt, pessimism, nihilistic thoughts, despair, hopelessness, agitation, self neglect, detachment or indifference
- Recovery from depression–increased physical energy with persisting depressed mood, recent discharge from hospital
- Availability of means of suicide–access to guns, isolated places

ABC of mental health

Management

When substantial mental disorder, such as depression, is present it should be treated adequately: the patient and his or her carers should be advised of potential side effects of drug treatment. With the patient's agreement, a few days' supply of drugs may be dispensed at a time. A specific appointment should be made for follow up assessment, and the patient and his or her carers should know whom to contact if matters deteriorate further.

Admission to hospital, under the Mental Health Act if necessary, may be the only realistic option. Hospital staff should be aware of the risks posed by a patient, and an appropriate level of vigilance maintained. Discharge plans should involve the carers, and take account of continued suicidal thoughts as other symptoms of depression subside and the patient regains his or her energy.

Violence

The best predictor of violence is a history of violent behaviour, and many potentially violent patients will have a documented forensic history. Men commit more violent acts than women, often within their family; violence to strangers is rare, and most perpetrators of violence are known to the victim. Drug or alcohol misuse is commonly associated with antisocial behaviour. The predictive value of any single risk factor is limited, and even assessments based on several factors are valid for only relatively short periods.

Although schizophrenia is the mental disorder most often associated with violence, the absolute risk in an individual patient is not high. Some personality disorders (especially those in cluster B— dissocial, impulsive, and emotionally unstable types, see Chapter 9), drug and alcohol misuse, and even depression may increase the risk of violence by a patient. Rarely, a patient with a phobic disorder (especially social phobia) may react aggressively if "trapped" or confined in a crowded place.

Assessment

As with the assessment of suicide risk, demographic factors associated with violence show poor specificity and sensitivity when applied to individual patients. The best predictors derive from a thorough knowledge of a patient's patterns of behaviour, habits, coping strategies, and tolerance of frustration, in conjunction with an evaluation of his or her mental state.

Although a personal history of violence is an important indicator of long term risk, it is the pattern and circumstances of such behaviour that is crucial to estimating risk in the short term. Changes in mental symptoms (such as intensifying persecutory delusions), behaviour (such as defaulting on treatment), or personal circumstances are particularly important.

Management

Management strategies depend on sharing information and responsibilities for monitoring among the clinical team. Important components are treating mental disorder, minimising the side effects of drugs, encouraging contact with services, assisting the patient in developing alternative coping techniques that avoid violence, and pre-empting situations in which violent behaviour is known to occur. Careful consideration should be given to warning carers of predicted risks and involving them in monitoring the patient's mental state.

Case history: Risk of dangerous behaviour associated with panic

Mr D, an 18 year old man with no history of psychiatric disorder, was encouraged by his girlfriend to take a ride on a big wheel at a fairground. While the wheel was in motion he experienced mild agitation, but attributed this to excitement. When the wheel stopped with his seat high above the ground, he was overwhelmed with panic and a desire to escape. He attempted to release his safety harness and jump out, and his girlfriend risked being dragged out as she tried to restrain him.

Feelings of panic subsided when the wheel started moving, and dissipated completely when he returned to the ground at the end of the ride. He could recall no similar experiences in the past, and has subsequently avoided great heights.

Demographic factors associated with high risk of violence

- Male
- Younger age
- History of aggressive or violent behaviour, especially involving weapons
- Personality disorder–especially dissocial or impulsive types, and those involving sadistic fantasies
- "Psychotic" mental illness–especially schizophrenia, morbid jealousy
- Alcohol or drug misuse
- "Organic" mental state–delirium, acute intoxication
- Unwillingness to accept treatment, or maintain contact with services

---

Patient factors associated with high risk of violence

- Threats or expressed intentions to harm someone
- Lack of regret or remorse for previous violence
- Delusions of passivity, control, jealousy, or of sexual interference.
- Delusions focused on particular people, especially if the patient feels threatened
- Hallucinations, especially of commands
- Agitation, which may be worsened by side effects of some drug treatments
- Inability to cope with stress or tolerate frustration, especially if associated with impulsive behaviour

---

Further reading

Appleby L. Panic and suicidal behaviour. *Brit J Psychiatry* 1994; 164:719-721.
Duggan C, ed. Assessing risk in the mentally disordered. *Brit J Psychiatry* 1997; 170 (suppl 32).
Calman KC, Royston GHD. Risk language and dialects. *BMJ* 1997;315:939-42.
Royal College of Psychiatrists. *Assessment and clinical management of risk of harm to other people.* London: RCPsych, 1996. (Council Report CR 53.)
Vincent C, ed. *Clinical risk management.* London: BMJ Publishing Group, 1995.
Westcott R. Emergencies, crises and violence. In: Pullen I, Wilkinson G, Wright A, Pereira Gray D, eds. *Psychiatry and general practice today.* London: Royal College of Psychiatrists and Royal College of General Practitioners, 1994: 170-179.

Index

Index

Index